MIGRAINE
RELIEF

MIGRAINE RELIEF

A Personal Treatment Program

Robert J. Kohlenberg, Ph.D.

HARPER & ROW, PUBLISHERS, New York
Cambridge, Philadelphia, San Francisco, London
1817 Mexico City, São Paulo, Sydney

To My Parents

Special thanks to Chuck Herring for his encouragement and ideas about publishing, to Tim Cahn for his able collaboration in the research, and to my patients who have taught me so much. No acknowledgment is complete without mentioning Mavis, who is wonderfully ever present in everything I do.

Published simultaneously in Great Britain by Harper & Row Limited, 28 Tavistock Street, London WC2E 7PN and in Australia and New Zealand by Harper & Row (Australasia) Pty. Limited, P.O. Box 226, Artarmon, New South Wales, 2064.

FIRST HARPER & ROW EDITION

Designer: C. Linda Dingler

Library of Congress Cataloging in Publication Data

Kohlenberg, Robert J.
    Migraine relief.
        1. Migraine—Treatment. 2. Biofeedback training.
1. Title.
RC392.K57 1983   616.8'5706   82-48233
ISBN 0-06-091026-7 (pbk) (U.S.A. and Canada)
    0-06-337032-8 (except U.S.A. and Canada)

83 84 85 86 87 10 9 8 7 6 5 4 3 2

CONTENTS

FOREWORD

The past few decades have seen an unprecedented advance in drug therapy of disease. It has been an important era, making available an impressive array of chemical compounds that have significantly increased both our understanding of diseases and our ability to treat them. Along with the very real benefits of these drugs has come the problem of unwanted side effects, which is inherent in drug therapy. Usually the side effects amount to minor nuisances, but sometimes they are serious and, rarely, calamities. Added to the known side effects is the realization that few, if any, medications have been in use long enough for us to know all the possible effects they may have in the body, especially when they are used for long periods of time. We are still discovering new properties, both good and bad, of aspirin, one of the oldest drugs in current medical use.

Given these problems with medications, it becomes understandable why many medical practitioners are enthusiastic (sometimes overly so) about biofeedback as a therapy that seems to offer an effectiveness comparable to drugs without the same potential for side effects. Biofeedback is not the panacea it is sometimes portrayed to be. Like all areas of medicine, there is still much to be learned. However, of all the physical problems that can be treated with this method, the treatment of headache has been the most consistently successful. Relaxation training, aided by biofeedback and stress management counseling, has added a powerful new tool for the control of both migraine and muscle-contraction headache, reducing or eliminating the need for medication in a large majority of patients.

Now, Dr. Robert Kohlenberg is presenting in this book a program in which the migraine sufferer can utilize temperature biofeedback and stress management techniques at home through self-instruction. It is, to my knowledge, a unique service and one that I believe will be useful to many people. In general, I do not think that self-help books can approach the effectiveness of working directly with a therapist. In this case, however, a special characteristic of the people who are prone to migraine seems to make this approach a good idea, i.e., they seem to be unusually motivated. I have been impressed with the diligence of most migraine patients in practicing the techniques they are taught. Assuming the user of this book has the same type of motivation, it will most likely result in significant improvement or complete relief.

I have been influenced to support the contents of this book in part by the fact that the material it contains has been tested in a special study to determine its effectiveness. The results indicate that it does work.

One word of warning: This book is written for a special type of person with a particular problem. That problem is migraine headache of either the classic or common vascular type. Many headaches that are assumed to be migraines aren't. If you have not already done so, check with your doctor to be sure of the diagnosis before embarking on the program. If, after consultation with your physician, you are satisfied that your headaches fit the description, then this approach deserves a trial. Good luck!

LYNDON E. LAMINACK, M.D.

PREFACE

When I began writing a self-help book for migraine headache sufferers, I was determined at the outset to evaluate the effectiveness of
the book. I did this by enlisting several hundred migraine sufferers
in the Seattle area. I cannot express my gratitude enough to these
subjects who for nearly one year sent in their weekly headache report forms which gave me information about the severity and number of headaches, as well as the amount of medication that they
used. A number of these subjects received this book (with one excep-
tion which I will describe later) which you are now reading. Other
subjects in the study received another book on headaches which is
widely available at bookstores and newsstands. That is, this book was
tested against a "control" book. I was pleased that *Migraine Relief*
was nearly three times as effective as the control book in helping
people overcome their migraine pain.

The letters that I have received from these subjects made my
efforts even more satisfying. Individuals who had suffered from
headaches for forty years and who have received nearly every type
of medical treatment were now nearly headache free. Other, young-
er individuals who had just started a family or career, whose lives
were seriously compromised by their headaches, also received benefit and expressed their gratitude.

Although my book was demonstrated scientifically to be effective, I was curious to find out how its usefulness could be increased.
To do this, I wrote to a number of subjects in the "control group"
who had reported improvement from reading the control book. Although the number of such individuals was much less than the number who improved from reading *Migraine Relief*, I thought perhaps
some new clues could be found to help migraine sufferers. I learned
that although the control book was several hundred pages long, most
of those subjects were helped by only one or two pages which discussed the role of food and migraine headaches. Again, although the

number of subjects helped was small, I was impressed by the effectiveness of certain diets in relieving migraine sufferers. This led me to study the whole area of food and food allergies and migraine headaches.

After thoroughly investigating the subject and attempting some of the techniques and diets on patients in my clinic, I became convinced that dietary factors could play a role for a significant number of migraine sufferers. The last chapter in this book, chapter 8, is devoted to this topic. I highly recommend that you read the first chapters before attempting the dietary regimen outlined in chapter 8. There is good reason to start with chapters 1 through 7 since most headaches can probably be relieved by these procedures alone. Further, the dietary factors discussed in chapter 8 are of little value unless you have learned the techniques and studied the information provided in the first seven chapters.

The purpose of this book is to make you aware of the progress of a migraine headache. The assessment of symptoms requires an expert. Proper diagnosis and therapy of all symptoms connected with migraine headaches, real or apparent, call for careful attention to your complaints by your doctor.

1

IS THIS BOOK FOR YOU?

If you are one of the 10 million migraine sufferers who are following their doctor's advice and still experiencing discomfort, this book is for you. It is very important, however, that you are sure that your headaches are wholly or partially of the migraine type. Only your doctor can give you this assurance. This book is for migraine or mixed (partial migraine) migraine or vascular headache sufferers who have seen their doctor and are under his/her care.

Symptoms of migraine

Migraine headaches include a wide variety of symptoms; thus they must be considered a complicated disorder. I have compiled a list of some of the complaints given by patients that have been associated with the diagnosis of migraine headaches. The first two complaints are the most common and usual symptoms, although you can be diagnosed as having migraine headaches without either of these symptoms present. Further, you can be given a completely different diagnosis even though you have these symptoms. The remaining complaints on the list are frequently reported by migraine sufferers but not nearly so often and consistently as these two.

The first and most common symptom is that the headache itself is located on either the right or the left side of the head. In fact, the word *migraine* is derived from an ancient diagnostic term, *hemicrania*, coined by one of the old Roman physicians, Galen. The term *hemicrania* became translated into the Italian *magrama*, and eventually into French as *migraine*. The original word *hemicrania* means "half a head." Usually a migraine *starts* on one side of the head but later can involve the entire head and other parts of the body. It might start on the left side one time, on the right side the other, although it is not uncommon for it always to start on one side for a particular patient. Usually the pain itself has a hammering, throbbing, or pushing quality, but some patients describe their pain as pressing and dull, burning, stretching, or pinpoint sharp. In one case, it was described as a nail being thrust into the head, deep into the brain itself.

The second symptom on this list, nausea, is also most commonly associated with migraine headaches. In some patients the nausea is slight and hardly noticeable, whereas in others, it is overpowering and may result in retching and vomiting. In the milder forms of nausea, my patients may not report any sick feeling but instead tell me that they stay away from food because they know that if they were to eat, they would most certainly become sick. Again, I want to emphasize that your migraine may involve both pain and nausea. Conversely, even though both of these symptoms are present, it may indicated a disorder other than migraine that needs to be appropriately treated. This is why it is so important for you to see your doctor to get an accurate diagnosis.

The other major type of headache that people experience is called *tension*, or muscle contraction, headache. These headaches are normally associated with excessive muscle contraction and have a set of symptoms slightly different from migraine headaches. Probably more often than not, headaches contain elements of both the tension and migraine types. It is therefore not unusual to have a diagnosis of mixed, or partial, migraine. This simply means that the discomfort you experience is the result of both a tension and a migraine headache.

The methods given in this book work perfectly well for both the pure and mixed migraine pain.

Symptom list

1. Pain on one side of the head. Almost any part of the head can be involved. Even though the pain begins on one side of the head it may move forward, backward, and involve the entire head. At times it may even move into the neck and shoulders.
2. Nausea. This includes a decided sick feeling that can result in retching and vomiting, as well as its more mild form in which the sight or thought of food is avoided.
3. Light sensitivity. Patients with this symptom prefer to remain in a darkened room.
4. Noise sensitivity. Noise levels easily tolerated during non-headache periods can become extremely irritating during an attack.
5. Chest or breastbone area pain. Although usually these

pains occur after the headache has started, in some cases these pains are the primary symptom of the migraine.

6. Marked change in facial color. This can either be a red or blushing appearance or a pale ashen color.

7. Eyes. Eyes may appear watery and/or bloodshot. Itching and burning might be experienced.

8. Nasal problems. Patients report either a stuffiness or runniness during the migraine attack.

9. Abdomen/bowel problems. During the course of the attack, an abdominal pain on the right side similar to appendicitis may be reported. Also a steady pain may radiate to the back. There may be constipation and/or diarrhea.

10. Lack of energy. A lack of motivation or lethargy all the way to extreme drowsiness can be a symptom of migraine.

11. Changes in mood. Most usually the patient who has mood changes associated with the migraine attack becomes very irritable, jumpy and extremely active, flitting about from one task to another. The opposite mood has also been experienced as part of an attack, i.e., depression, hopelessness, and misery.

12. Pains in other parts of the body. Almost every part of the body has been reported by some patients as the location of a migraine pain.

13. Hallucinations and other sensory disturbances that can involve vision, sense of touch, and other senses. Symptoms typically occur before the actual headache or pain phase of the migraine. These, and most of the other symptoms in the above list, are called "aura" when they precede or serve as warning signals that an actual migraine attack is about to begin. The symptoms may be as simple as blind spots, brilliant lights, sparks or flashes in geometric forms that appear before the eyes. The hallucination can also be well-developed visions of specific people or objects. Some patients report that people look as if they have halos around them. Many of the characters in Lewis Carroll's *Alice in Wonderland* are similar to the visual hallucinations experienced by some migraine sufferers. It is generally believed that Mr. Carroll did suffer from migraine headaches and experienced such auras.

Can you really stop your migraine headaches?

If you read this book and follow the directions contained on these pages, the chances are very good that you can stop or greatly reduce the pain of your migraine headaches. Probably you have already tried all kinds of treatments, each time hoping that you have finally found the cure for your headaches and each time being disappointed. All of these negative experiences and false promises can easily produce a cynical and closed mind. The ideas that I discuss on the following pages are new and sometimes startling. I'm not asking you to accept these ideas outright—just to keep an open mind so that you can give this approach a fair chance. I challenge the openness of your mind with the following statement:

In order to stop your headaches, you must learn to control the opening and closing of the blood vessels in your head.

Okay, I am aware of the confusion that this idea must produce in you. Almost everyone who reads this statement is going to ask, "How can I ever possibly learn how to control the opening and closing of the blood vessels in my head, and what does that have to do with my headaches?" Let me repeat that I am just asking you to be open to this idea and not to reject it categorically. Read further and find out why I think your headaches are caused by the opening up and closing down of your blood vessels. Then I will give you specific step-by-step instruction on how—with the aid of biofeedback and other techniques—you can gain control over the opening up and closing down of the blood vessels in your head.

First, however, we are going to have a look at the physiological and medical causes of your headaches. It is important to understand how your body works to produce headaches in order to see why it is necessary to learn how to change the activity of the blood vessels in your head.

Before we begin our tour of the body, I want to make a comment about the medical and scientific words used throughout this book. I strongly believe that everyday language is perfectly adequate to explain almost anything, and I, therefore, have avoided complicated, technical terms. There are however three medical terms that I think are very important and would like you to learn: *artery*, *vasoconstriction*, and *vasodilation*. These three terms form the core of understanding your migraine headaches.

Vasoconstriction and vasodilation

Here are some basic facts about your body. Your brain, like any other part of your body, needs blood to function properly; it needs more or less blood depending upon the task at hand. For the blood to get up to the brain it has to pass through a system of muscular tubes, or pipes, called *arteries*. The arteries have the ability to open and close, letting more or less blood pass through them.

Your blood vessels are not lazy. In fact they are constantly changing size, depending in part on what's going on inside, as well as around you. If I quietly sneak up behind you and suddenly clap my hands, the arteries in your body will automatically react—some of them will open up and some will close down. Thus, more or less blood will flow to various regions in the body. There will be vasodilation and vasoconstriction. (The *a-s* in *vasoconstriction* and *vasodilation* is pronounced just like the *ays* in d*ays*.)

Vaso means blood vessels, whereas *constriction* refers to something squeezed together or restrained. Thus, *vasoconstriction* means the closing down of an artery so that it restricts the flow of blood. *Dilation*, on the other hand, refers to something that has been opened up or made larger. *Vasodilation*, then, means the opening up of an artery to allow a larger amount of blood to flow through.

What happens to your arteries when I sneak up behind you and suddenly clap my hands? If you are frightened by the sudden noise, an automatic pattern of artery changes will take place. The arteries in your hands will close down, or vasoconstrict. The arteries leading to your brain will also close down, or vasoconstrict. Arteries in other regions will also change, but I want to focus on those arteries in your hands and in your brain: You have a very reactive group of arteries which feed blood to your brain, as well as to the rest of your body.

Blood vessels run amok: a real pain

A migraine headache always begins with vasoconstriction in your head. The arteries close down to a very great extent, letting just a small amount of blood up into your brain. At the same time that the arteries are closing down in your head, the arteries in your hands are also closing down. Although vasoconstriction is a very normal biological process, people with migraine headaches probably show this more often and to a greater degree than other people. Interestingly enough, the closing down of your arteries does not produce pain, but it might produce an aura, the warning signal that a headache is about to start. In some people, it can consist of a visual hallucination, an odor, a bright flashing light, lethargy, etc. Auras are quite an interesting aspect of the migraine headache, though it is perfectly normal and quite common for migraine sufferers never to experience one.

If the closing down of your arteries, or vasoconstriction, is not what produces the pain, what does? The pain comes from a very logical response of your body to the reduced blood supply to your brain. All of us have a built-in biological thermostat to correct extreme states in any of our bodily functions. If you are doing a lot of hard physical work on a hot day, the thermostat within your body senses that the body temperature is going up. To compensate and bring your body temperature down, it brings into play a number of mechanisms, including sweating. Similarly, the migraine sufferer who has been subjected to vasoconstriction brings into play a thermostatic mechanism which tends to correct for the constriction by opening up, or vasodilating, the arteries. Unfortunately, this corrective mechanism in the migraine sufferer's body overdoes its job. It opens the arteries too fast, too far, and leaves them open—wide open—too long. It is during the opened up portion of this reaction that you experience the severe pain of the migraine. The reason that medication, such as ergotamine, is sometimes effective is because these substances constrict the arteries, thus eliminating the source of the pain. For many patients, however, the side effects of the medications are uncomfortable and too long lasting, and these patients are generally hesitant about using the drugs.

Above all, it is important to remember that a migraine headache involves arteries in the head and a sequence of two reactions. The first reaction is vasoconstriction, a closing down of the arteries. The second reaction is the body's attempt to compensate by vasodilating, which it does too much. The pain of the migraine is experienced during this second reaction.

Why you overvasodilate

The processes of vasoconstriction and then the corrective reaction of your body to cause vasodilation are normal processes that occur in every person. The problem is that you, the migraine sufferer, probably overrespond with constrictions and do so more frequently and to a larger extent than most other people. Similarly, you probably at times overcompensate and dilate too much after the constriction has occurred.

Why does this happen in your body whereas it doesn't happen in others? This question is really difficult to answer since many factors could account for the difference between you and individuals who do not suffer from migraine headaches. To begin with, there is strong evidence that people tend to differ in their physiological reactions to the everyday stresses and strains that we all encounter.

Consider the simple experiment that I described earlier, in which I suddenly clap my hands to produce changes in the opening and closing of arteries within your body. Other changes occur in other bodily systems at the same time that your arteries react. There will be a change in heartbeat, respiration, sweat gland activity, the flow of digestive juices, breathing rate, brain rhythm. That is, even a stimulus as mild as a handclap produces a host of bodily changes in every person.

Not everybody, however, reacts to the same extent in each of these bodily systems. For some people, their heartbeat may show a marked change, whereas arteries, sweat gland activity, etc., may show relatively small changes. Other individuals may show an extremely large increase in sweat gland activity whereas all of the other bodily systems change only a small amount. Each person seems to be endowed with a unique reactive bodily system. For this reason some people tend to have symptoms like excessive acid in the stomach when they have experienced too much stress whereas others may show heart problems in reaction to the same stress. I am suggesting that you just happen to have the kind of body that is extremely reactive in its arterial system, which then makes you prone to migraine.

This, of course, suggests that you may have inherited this tendency to have overreactive arteries from your parents. It is well known that migraine headaches tend to run in families. For example, if one parent has migraine, the chances are four out of ten that the children will also suffer from these headaches. If both parents have migraine, the chances go up to seven out of ten that the children will follow in kind.

There are other indications that a migraine sufferer tends to be particularly prone to overreactive arteries. It is not uncommon for women who regularly experience severe migraine pain to have this pain disappear during pregnancy. Extensive changes in hormones occur during pregnancy which probably have a lot to do with the disappearance of the headaches. It is unknown whether pregnancy produces hormones that make up for a deficiency during nonpregnant times in the woman's life or whether there is no deficiency but certain biochemicals necessary for the development of the fetus produce an extraordinary protective response.

Some migraine sufferers only experience their headaches once a month in relation to their menstrual cycles. Again, this shows that these patients are probably not overreactive with their arterial system during most of the month but due to the biochemical changes that occur on a monthly basis, become vulnerable to overreactive arteries and the resulting migraine pain.

Although all of the above suggests that there is a strong physical basis for the migraine syndrome, one really cannot conclude that the migraines are caused by genetic or hormonal factors. It is more accurate to say that these factors tend to make an individual susceptible to overreactive arteries but do not cause the overreaction itself. In most cases, migraine headaches are probably caused by a combination of the individual's susceptibility and the stresses and strains of everyday living.

Migraine headaches are probably caused by a combination of the individual's susceptibility and the stresses and strains of everyday living.

In any event, I feel strongly that you can learn how to control and stop your headaches. There is a great deal you can do about the immediate cause of your headaches—vasoconstrictions followed by the painful overvasodilations.

What you can do about the cause of your headaches

In order to avoid migraines, you must learn how to prevent overvasodilation. My plan to help you do this is quite straightforward, although I admit that at first it might sound difficult. There are two parts to your attack on migraine pain. The first is to prevent, as much as possible, constriction of the arteries in your head. These constrictions are the body's first step in the two-step reaction that leads to migraine pain. The second part of your migraine prevention plan concerns what to do once your arteries have constricted. Both parts of this migraine prevention plan are explained in the remaining pages of this book. Let's begin by discussing what can be done about constricted arteries.

First learn to gently open up the arteries in your head at will.

Once you have constricted arteries in your head, I would like you to voluntarily dilate your arteries in a gentle, normal, relaxed manner rather that waiting for the body and its thermostatic mechanism to do an overkill job. Thus, the first skill I ask you to learn in order to stop your headaches is how to gently open up the arteries in your head at will, without the use of drugs.

In the next chapter, entitled "Biofeedback" you will learn how to use the temperature sensitive, or biotic, band on your finger to teach yourself voluntary control over your arteries. Once you have learned to do this, you will have learned a great deal about how to get rid of your headaches, and you will be able to avoid a considerable amount of pain.

Why do you insist on constricting your arteries in the first place?

The reasons for the vasoconstriction and the overcompensating dilation are best understood when you consider that our bodies are designed for living in the forest. It is only relatively recently in the history of humankind that we have lived in the safety and security of our homes. When we want to eat, we don't have to look for animals to kill; we simply walk to the local hamburger stand or grocery store. We don't have to carry weapons to protect ourselves from antagonistic neighbors. Our bodies, however, are exquisitely constructed to enable us, in fact, to hunt our own food, fight wild animals, and protect ourselves physically from the aggression of our neighbors.

Imagine yourself living ten thousand years ago in a rich and fertile forest. You are happily walking along a path; suddenly a ferocious tiger leaps out from behind some bushes and begins to race at you, growling and drooling. Your remarkable body automatically gets you ready for this significant event. Your heart begins to beat faster, adrenalin is pumped into your blood vessels, and very interesting curious changes occur in the arteries in your body.

During this process, the arteries in your hands, in your feet, in your legs and near the surface of the skin constrict. After all, you might get bitten, and a superficial wound richly served by normally functioning arteries would result in excessive bleeding. Too much bleeding could, in turn, result in premature weakness and death. Getting ready to fight or run from the tiger is not a time for high-level thinking, planning, and calculating. You don't need a highly tuned, active brain at this point. You simply need to coordinate your muscles to either run or fight. Since you need muscles and not your brain, the arteries leading up to your brain close down (constrict) and carry blood away from the brain. This reaction, plus the constriction of the arteries serving the surface of hands and other extremities, allows more blood to be directed toward the deep organs and muscles. These deeper muscles will definitely be needed to run from or fight with the tiger. A good supply of blood to these muscles is essential and perhaps could determine whether you will live or die.

Let's say that (1) the fight with your tiger or flight from him continued for a fairly long period of time; (2) arteries leading to your brain are constricted during the time that this fighting or running goes on; and (3) you have a faulty thermostatic mechanism that will attempt to overcome and compensate for these closed-down arteries. So, when the fight or flight is over, and perhaps even before, you will have a terrible, splitting migraine.

What caused your migraine these thousands of years ago? It started with the appearance of the tiger, which produced a very normal, adaptive, and essential change in the blood vessels leading to your brain and to the other parts of your body. The next thing that happened was the blood vessels to your brain became constricted for a long period of time. Finally, when you had a chance to rest, your faulty thermostat opened your brain arteries so wide and kept them open for so long that you had a full-blown migraine. It is interesting to note that many current-day migraines occur during restful times, like on weekends, after work, after the company has left.

Of course, not all headaches occur in the "rest" period after the danger has gone away. Migraines can come on just as easily at almost any point after the initial constriction has occurred. For some people, even the smallest constriction present for only a half-hour or so can trigger the automatic thermostat that produces a painful vasodilation. For other patients, the vasoconstriction can be around for days, and since the thermostat has not yet tried to correct this condition, the headache pain is not experienced. Interestingly, the same individuals can sometimes withstand long-term vasoconstrictions that should result in headaches, but, at other times, a brief constriction can almost immediately trigger a painful overdilation. I have often observed this latter pattern in women who tend to get migraines during their menstrual cycle.

It is interesting to note that many current-day migraines occur during restful times, like on weekends, after work, after the company has left.

"Okay," you say, "that seems to make sense." Chances are, however, that as you can best remember, the migraine you had a week ago didn't start with a ferocious tiger suddenly confronting you. In fact, you can assure me that you have never had a migraine which was caused by a tiger. Instead, as one patient with a twenty-year history of severe migraines told me, "The very first headache I had came right after a visit from my new mother-in-law, who I so terribly wanted to impress with my clean house."

You probably understand where I am headed. Instead of getting ready to fight a tiger, you are using your most exquisitely designed, complicated body to fight or run from your mother-in-law, your dirty living room, your child who is in trouble at school, your spouse who gets angry at you, your speeding ticket, your examination, your report that is due tomorrow, your employee who is not doing a good enough job, your boss who gave you a poor evaluation, etc., etc., etc. Your forest person's body reacts to all of these and a myriad other stressors that occur in daily life in a manner appropriate to the forest and not to the city.

To make matters even worse, your body is reacting in a way that actually prevents you from dealing most effectively with the problems that confront you. If you recall, when your arteries constrict, you are not getting sufficient blood into your brain so it can operate efficiently and cleverly. The higher-thinking centers of your brain barely get enough blood to solve ordinary problems, such as whether to run or fight or climb a tree. Just imagine your blood-depleted brain trying to process and handle complicated problems, such as financial management, child rearing, or interpersonal crises. Not only are you giving yourself a migraine, but you are not using all your resources to solve your problems, either.

As a professor, I often had the chance to observe first-hand the effects of vasoconstriction on poor mental functioning. After every exam, I invariably would be visited by several students who told me that they diligently studied and knew the material inside and out but their minds went blank when the exams were placed on their desks. They just couldn't think and hence performed poorly. I now know why they couldn't think. Those students reacted to the exam as though it were a tiger. Their bodies automatically diverted blood into the deeper muscles, and there simply wasn't enough blood getting to their brains.

Your body is reacting in a way that actually prevents you from dealing most effectively with the problems that confront you.

What you can do about those "tigers"

Chapters 5 and 6 in this book discuss how to stop seeing those blood vessel-constricting tigers around every corner. There are good techniques that allow you to use your intelligence to analyze problems in a way that will overcome the natural reactions of the vascular system in your body which lead to so much trouble.

Have you ever noticed that some people react to a problem as though it were the end of the world, whereas to you, that same problem doesn't seem to be important? I have a patient who was greatly distressed over the fact that he had only a hundred thousand dollars inheritance with which to invest and plan his future. "If only I had two hundred thousand," he said, "I could put it into tax-free bonds and make enough money to live off the interest. It's just driving me crazy to find the very best way to get the most out of this inadequate sum of money." His problem resulted in a series of migraine headaches.

You wish you had such problems? Even though my patient reacted to his problem as though it were a ferocious tiger, most of you would probably feel it would be more of a joy and a delight than a stress. The difference between you and my patient is in the way you analyze the problem confronting you.

My patient saw his problem of "insufficient" money as a danger signal to which his body responded. When considering those items that are danger signals to you and not somebody else, the difference between you and that other person is also the difference in the way you think about and analyze the problem. If you want to learn how to stop that vasoconstriction from occurring in the first place, it would be desirable for you to learn some new ways of analyzing your problems.

If you want to learn how to stop that vasoconstriction from occurring in the first place, it would be desirable for you to learn some new ways of analyzing your problems.

A great many of the stresses that we respond to in our daily lives can be avoided. You can stay away from them, but it takes special skills and real determination to do so. I am not saying that you can run away from the world and the problems around you. I am saying that you can learn how to pace your life and structure it so that you are not constantly under stress.

Consider the following patient of mine who didn't avoid a tiger when she could have. As is true for many of my migraine patients, Clara had a very busy life. In addition to taking complete responsibility for cleaning and managing a large home, making sure her four children were clothed and fed, being a good wife and companion to her overworked husband, Clara also worked full-time as a teacher. Periodically she had to turn in rather complicated reports on her various classroom activities. She had planned to use the weekend for preparing these tedious, yet required, reports that were due the following Monday. Unexpectedly, some out-of-town friends called up stating that they were in town and would like to come over and have dinner and spend the weekend with Clara and her family. Rather than saying, "No, I only have time to have cake and coffee with you," Clara outwardly sounded excited and jubilant and asked them to come over immediately. After she hung up the phone she looked around the house and saw the mess that it was in. She had previously started a simple dinner for her family and now realized she would have to make something much more elaborate and larger. Bang! Down went the blood vessels in her head, which incidentally stayed closed for most of the weekend until her thermostatic mechanism finally put her in bed with one of the worst migraines she had ever experienced. She did not get the reports done on time. In fact, she fell considerably behind in her reporting and household chores because she was unable to return to work for the rest of that week. If only she had said no she wouldn't have created the stressful situation that triggered her migraine.

Although this is an extreme example, much milder forms may occur almost daily for you. I will tell you how to change your yes saying behaviors so that you can stay away from many of the stress-producing situations we create for ourselves.

Taking care of your arteries

Now you know what this book is about. It is about the proper care and feeding of the arteries in your head. You are going to learn how to open them up through the use of biofeedback in a very gentle and painless way. You are also going to change some of the ways you analyze problems so that your arteries will stop closing down so often and so tightly in reaction to your daily problems and stresses. You will learn how to defuse all those bombs lying in the outside world that now explode so often and stop the blood from getting into your head. Finally, you will discover how to avoid having to expose yourself unnecessarily to some stresses and strains that you now confront which trigger vasoconstriction.

> You are going to change some of the ways you analyze problems so that your arteries will stop closing down so often and so tightly.

How to use this book

Read this book at your own pace. Each of the following chapters will have some specific suggestions to help you overcome and prevent migraine pain. In the following pages you will learn some new skills, each of which will form a part of the overall goal of allowing you to be master of your arteries. In a way, each of the tasks and suggestions can be likened to the various colors that an artist uses in creating a painting. Each time a new color is added to the canvas, it not only makes the painting more complete, but enhances the colors that have already been brushed on. Each color by itself is important and does part of the job: The greens for leaves on a tree can convey the feeling of the leaf. Additions of blue for the sky and browns for the hills not only make the painting more complete but enhance the vividness and clarity of the green originally used for the leaves.

As you acquire and add the new skills that I discuss in this book, each will enhance and make more complete your shield against unnecessary migraine pain.

Some people may wish to get an overall idea of the picture before they begin actually working on the parts. If you are so inclined, read through the whole book before you actually begin practicing the various techniques. On the other hand, the chapters are arranged in a step-by-step sequence so that you may read at your leisure and try the suggestions as they come up.

There is no fixed time schedule or rate for reading this book. The important thing is that you feel comfortable with the concepts presented and have a good understanding of the skills described. As your painting becomes more and more complete, so too will your control of headaches.

2

BIOFEEDBACK–USING THE BIOTIC BAND

Please read this chapter carefully. I start with this request because curiosity about biofeedback and the use of the biotic band could easily tempt the reader to skip over details in order to begin biofeedback as soon as possible. A desire to start doing something about migraine pain could also lead you to skip ahead before you have learned some of the basics required for success.

Try to be patient.

In order to learn how to counteract your constricted arteries, you should go methodically through this chapter step by step. It is important that you thoroughly understand the whys and the why nots of biofeedback training and its application to stopping the onset of a migraine headache. As you progress through this chapter, you will be learning the skills that will form the cornerstone of your personal migraine treatment program.

Let's being with the goals of this particular chapter. The overall goal is, of course, to learn how to stop the early stages of a migraine headache and thus prevent the occurrence of the headache itself. I emphasize the *preventive approach* used in this chapter and throughout this book. The skills learned in this chapter are to be used by you *before* the headache itself starts. All our attention is focused on counteracting the vasoconstriction which occurs before the headache pain. This is done by *voluntary vasodilation*.

After you have learned how to vasodilate, you should regularly practice a vasodilation exercise during the day. Further, I would like you to use your dilation skills to gently open up arteries whenever you are aware that they have become constricted. These two activities can be compared to the preventive measures you take with an automobile. The first, regularly performing a vasodilation exercise during the day, is like giving your car regular lubrication even though everything seems to be working just fine. The second process,

> The overall goal is to learn how to stop the early stages of a migraine headache and thus prevent the occurrence of the headache itself.

dilating arteries whenever you become aware that they are constricting, is like lubricating your car when you hear a squeaking noise but no serious damage has yet taken place.

Before you can take these preventive measures, however, you must learn how to gain voluntary control over the blood vessels in your head and be able to gently dilate them at will. In order to accomplish this overall goal, I will give you step-by-step instructions on the use of the biotic band which is a biofeedback device. The biotic band can help you learn to voluntarily increase your finger temperature by helping you learn to control the arteries that supply blood to your hands and fingers.

I know that your headache does not occur in your hands and that head pain is not caused by vasoconstrictions and dilations in your fingers. There are logical reasons, however, for asking you to learn to control your finger temperature even though we are really interested in having you voluntarily control the arteries in your head.

There appears to be a direct relationship between the arteries in your head and the vasoconstrictions and vasodilations in your hand. Learning to control the arteries in your hands will automatically produce the desired changes in your head. This is a very convenient state of affairs because the arteries in your head are quite inaccessible and do not readily lend themselves to measurement and biofeedback training. The correlation between arteries in both places, however, does make possible the use of biofeedback devices that are easily attached and removed. The reason that the temperature of your fingers is directly related to the amount of vasodilation and constriction that occurs is that warmth depends upon the amount of blood flowing through the arteries. If your arteries are open and allow blood to pass through easily, then the warmth of your hand will increase. Conversely, if your arteries begin to constrict, then the amount of blood flowing through your fingers will decrease and the temperature will also decrease.

The whole idea of *learning* how to *voluntarily* control vasoconstrictions and vasodilations in order to prevent migraines still astounds me. That such voluntary control can be learned, as well as its clinical importance in terms of migraine pain, was discovered by researchers at the Menninger Clinic in the early 1970s. They found that migraine sufferers who had learned how to raise their hand temperatures (through biofeedback training in the clinic laboratories) were able to abort or prevent migraine headaches from occurring in the outside world by using this skill of handwarming whenever they felt that they might be getting a migraine headache. These patients were delighted with the results and served as a stimulus that launched a decade of research into the mechanisms and processes involved in this revolutionary treatment.

What is biofeedback?

The principle involved in biofeedback is so basic that we usually take it for granted: Given a goal we are striving for, we need to know how successful our efforts are toward reaching that goal in order to alter our activities as necessary.

Imagine how much harder it would be, for example, to hit a baseball with a bat if you were blindfolded. You'd swing and miss. How would you change your next swing to improve your chances for a hit? Were you high? low? close?

When you attempt to dilate the arteries in your hands, you have no way of telling if your method is working—no way to see whether you need to modify or change your approach. The biotic band shows you the results of your efforts; it gives you the information you need to be successful.

The biotic band

I would like to point out that I interchange the terms "warm your hands" with "vasodilate arteries to your hands" and "vasodilate arteries to your head." Basically, all these terms are functionally equivalent; when you say one, it implies the other two.

In using the biotic band to prevent migraines, keep in mind that a vasoconstriction in your head occurs at the same time as a constriction in your fingers. Similarly, head dilations occur at the same time as finger dilations; thus once you have learned how to dilate finger arteries, you automatically know how to dilate the arteries in your head.

Once you have learned to dilate finger arteries, you automatically then know how to dilate the arteries in your head.

It is important to remember that the warmth or the temperature of your finger is related to the amount of blood flowing through it. Therefore, if your hands are cool, it means that the arteries are constricted; if your hands are warm, they are vasodilated. Our primary concern is to prevent vasoconstriction by keeping your hands as warm as possible and to reverse the effects of a vasoconstriction by warming your hands once they have started to cool off. Using your biotic band will teach you how to increase the temperature of your fingers.

Using your biotic band will teach you how to increase the temperature of your fingers.

Incidentally, there is a vast difference between the temperature of your fingers and the core temperature of your body. The latter is obtained by placing a thermometer under your tongue and is a very useful diagnostic tool for detecting illnesses. Core temperature only varies a few degrees from 98.6 degrees.

Your finger temperature, on the other hand, can show swings as much as 25 degrees one way or the other. Therefore, do not become alarmed if you find, for example, that your finger temperature is less than 78 degrees, the lowest temperature that your biotic band can measure. In fact, many migraine people do have relatively cool hands and feet most of the time. On the other hand, there are many migraine sufferers who seem to have relatively warm hands most of the time.

There are great individual differences in the finger temperatures of migraine sufferers. I have also observed, among my patients, great differences in the amount of hand temperature drop or increase when vasoconstriction or vasodilation occurs. You might find your hand temperature to be quite variable with readings of 78 degrees or lower at one time and 90 degrees or above at another time.

The temperature changes in your own hands from time to time may reflect the vasodilation or constriction that is present, but they may also reflect the temperature of the room in which you happen to be using the biotic band. So unless the temperature of the room remains fairly constant, I would recommend caution in interpreting the actual reading of finger temperature from one week to the next as being solely due to vasodilation or vasoconstriction.

However, the most important use of the biotic band will not be to measure your finger temperature from one week to the next, but *from one minute to the next*. Since it is unlikely that the room temperature is going to change within a few minutes, changes in temperature on your biotic band within a few minutes' time are definite indications of vasodilation or vasoconstriction and not changes in room temperature.

When you learn how to vasodilate arteries, the initial conditions might vary considerably from time to time. Under some conditions, your initial hand temperature might be 90 degrees; at other times, your hand temperature might be 81 degrees. In either events, the dilation skills that you have learned will allow you to increase your finger temperature even though the *amount* of increase you can expect is quite different in these two situations. If your initial hand temperature is as high as 90 degrees, it would be extremely difficult to elevate your temperature more than a few degrees beyond that point. Whereas if your temperature is considerably lower, you might find that you can raise your temperature 10 or even 15 degrees when you apply your vasodilation skills.

What I am saying here is: We are more interested in the *process* by which you change your temperature, regardless of its initial reading, than the actual value of the reading or the amount of change. This does not mean, however, that there is no useful information in your initial or actual temperature reading because as you gain more and more experience in being aware of your actual finger temperature, you will learn to interpret it in a meaningful way.

Now, let us begin to use the biotic band to measure vasoconstriction as indicated by finger temperature.

Learning to read the biotic band

It is most important that you learn how to accurately read your biotic band. This is critical to your learning how to control blood vessels. Reading the biotic band is a little tricky, so make sure you have mastered the next section before moving on.

Place the biotic band in front of you, flat on the table. You will notice two rows of printed numbers. These numbers are in degrees Fahrenheit. You can also see that at the bottom of the band the lowest number is 78 degrees Fahrenheit. Similarly the top of the band shows 96 degrees. This means that if the temperature of your finger is above 98 degrees (it will soon be apparent why I have said 98 degrees rather than 96 degrees) you will not be able to use the biotic band as a precision biofeedback device at this time. In a few minutes you will be ready to take the initial finger temperature, and if you find that the biotic band is not adequate to measure your temperature, don't get upset. I have included a section at the end of this chapter on just this state of affairs.

Beside each number on the biotic band is a square area which is not visible at this time (as long as the room temperature is less than 78 degrees). Each one of these dots contains a liquid crystal substance which changes color as the temperature of your finger changes. Liquid crystal is the same substance that was used in the "mood" rings so popular a few years ago. The squares can either be the color they are now, a deep almost black hue, or as the temperature increases change in color from red-tan to orange to yellow-green to blue-green and finally to a solid blue color. By reading the highest square that is illuminated across from one of the numbers on the band, you can make a fairly accurate determination of your finger temperature as shown in the table below.

BIOTIC BAND TEMPERATURE TABLE

LIGHTED DEGREE	RED-TAN	ORANGE	YELLOW-GREEN	BLUE-GREEN	BLUE
78°	78°	78.5°	79°	79.5°	80°
80°	80°	80.5°	81°	81.5°	82°
82°	82°	82.5°	83°	83.5°	84°
84°	84°	84.5°	85°	85.5°	86°
86°	86°	86.5°	87°	87.5°	88°
88°	88°	88.5°	89°	89.5°	90°
90°	90°	90.5°	91°	91.5°	92°
92°	92°	92.5°	93°	93.5°	94°
94°	94°	94.5°	95°	95.5°	96°
96°	96°	96.5°	97°	97.5°	98°

Always read the highest temperature showing and ignore the purple color which may sometimes be visible on some squares.

Both the number next to the square as well as the color of the square is used to determine the degrees Fahrenheit temperature reading. You can now see how it is possible to read a temperature at 98 degrees even though the highest number on the band is 96 degrees. If the highest square illuminated on the biotic band is next to the 96 degrees mark and if the color of the square is blue, the actual temperature, as shown in the table, is 98 degrees. Similarly, you can read temperatures in half degree steps by using the number and color of the square. For example, if the highest square illuminated is next to the 78 degrees mark and if the square is orange, the actual temperature is 78.5 degrees.

Do these two experiments

The following two experiments will help you to become familiar with reading the biotic band. Remember, you must be able to read the temperature indicated on the biotic band before it can be used for biofeedback. The first experiment will just take a few seconds.

Hold the band up to your mouth and breathe warm air over the face for several seconds. This will activate the liquid crystal squares on your band. Now move the band away so that you can see the squares change color quite rapidly as they begin to cool off. You will notice that the highest square that is illuminated will reverse backward through the color range shown on the table until it is no longer showing any color and the square below it will go through the same color change sequence. These color changes occur so rapidly, however, that you might not be able to see all the colors distinctly.

Next take three ordinary water glasses. Fill one of them half full with tepid water. The water should be about as warm as your forehead but almost any temperature will do as long as it is in the lukewarm range. Fill the other two glasses with very cold water in one and very hot water in the other. Now use two pieces of Scotch tape to attach the biotic band to the outside of the lower part of the lukewarm glass, making sure that the numbers are easily readable, that the back of the numbered face is flat against the glass, and that the cellophane tape does not cover the numbers or squares.

If none of the squares is illuminated, the water is either too cold or too hot. Add small amounts of either cold or hot water until a square or squares are illuminated. Practice using the table to read the temperature. Now, by adding a very small amount of warm water, get the squares to change color so that it reads one-half degree higher. Make the square change up and down through the color range so that you can see what red-tan, orange, yellow-green, blue-green and blue actually look like. Remember, always use the highest temperature shown for your reading; ignore other lower temperature squares that might be illuminated.

After you are confident that you can read the biotic band, you are ready to try it on your finger.

Placing the biotic band on your finger

The biotic band should be loosely wrapped around your finger so that the face of the band is on the pad of your finger and not on the nail side. The band should be arranged so that, as you sit and look at your palms-up hand, you can read the numbers in their right-side-up position.

The main mistake that people make at this point is attaching the biotic band too tightly. Remember, the temperature indicates the amount of blood flowing into the finger, and it is quite easy to constrict this flow by having the band on too tightly. It should be on loosely enough so that you can easily remove it without having to undo the velcro strips. If you ever feel any throbbing or your finger changes color while the band is in place, you know that the band is on too tightly.

It is also important that you use the band on the same finger and in the same position each time you use it. I suggest that you use the left index finger, although this is optional and you can use any finger that seems most comfortable for you. Once the band is in the right position and not on too tightly, you are ready to take your first finger temperature reading. Remember to (1) ignore any of the very dark blue that may be illuminated; (2) always use the highest temperature reading as your actual finger temperature.

Take your reading now. If your hand temperature is less than 78 degrees, you will not get a reading on your biotic band. Do not be alarmed, this is normal and is discussed later in this chapter. Once you have determined what your finger temperature is, write it down along with the date and time. It is good practice to keep records of your finger temperature in your experimentation with biofeedback. I have included a personal handwarming diary in the back of this book, and I highly recommend that you use it. You can begin using the diary right now by recording the finger temperature you have just taken.

Your first attempt to dilate arteries

Leave the biotic band in place on your finger. In a few moments, I'm going to ask you to settle back in a comfortable position, close your eyes, and tell yourself the word "vasodilate." I would then like you to try doing whatever you think might vasodilate your arteries and increase your finger temperature. I do not expect you to know what to do at this point, but I would like you to experiment, using whatever you think is going to help warm your hands. Give it a try for three or four minutes, then open your eyes and immediately read the temperature on the band.

Try it now.

After you've tried it, record the temperature reading alongside the first or beginning temperature that you recorded. Find the difference between the second, or "after," reading and the first, or "before," reading. What you are doing with the biotic band is teaching yourself how to raise your finger temperature as much as possible within a three- or four-minute period of time. Once you can do this on a reliable basis, you will have gained voluntary control over the arteries supplying blood to your hand and you will then automatically be able to control the arteries supplying blood to your head.

A number of things may have happened during this initial biofeedback trial. First, there may have been no change whatsoever in the temperature of your finger as a result of your efforts. This indicates that whatever you tried to do was not effective or at least was not effective when tried this first time. Second, your temperature may have increased, showing that whatever you're doing is at least a step in the right direction and should be elaborated on or improved upon in additional practice sessions. Finally, your temperature may have dropped. This temperature drop may be due to the fact that you were trying too hard. That is, you were approaching this task of attempting to dilate your arteries as though it were a challenge.

One of the things I can tell you *not* to do during your biofeedback attempt is to approach it as a challenge and something that must be overcome. You will find that the harder you try the less successful you will be. It is best to sit back and take a very nonchalant or casual attitude toward the whole thing. For many of my patients that particular instruction gives them the most difficulty. They're just not sure how to take a nonchalant attitude and let something happen.

Sit back and take a very nonchalant or casual attitude toward the whole thing.

I see this difficulty particularly in successful executives who have been well rewarded for their many years of hard, driving effort and their ability to "make things happen." I have often seen such patients seated in the chair with the biofeedback device attached to their finger, their eyes closed, and their fingers and knuckles white from tightly clenching the chair in their efforts to make their finger temperature increase. Such efforts, of course, only result in vasoconstriction and decreased blood flow and drops in finger temperature.

Finding out whether or not your finger temperature stayed the same, increased, or decreased during your first attempt is what biofeedback is all about. You can use this information about what happened to your finger temperature (biofeedback) to guide your future efforts.

Practice, practice, practice

Carry your biotic band with you at all times. Try to use it at least four times throughout the day. It only takes a few minutes to do one biofeedback learning session. Each time you practice, say the word "vasodilate" to yourself and try to raise your temperature in a three- to four-minute period. Be persistent and eventually your efforts will be rewarded. Use the diary and record your "before" and "after" temperature for each of these three- to four-minute biofeedback experiments. As you practice, you are learning a precise skill that will help you to avoid a migraine.

> The more you practice, the faster you will learn how to control your migraines.

The number of days that it takes to learn how to control your arteries through the use of the biotic band can vary considerably from person to person. Good control over arteries, which means that there is a reliable increase in temperature, even though it is a small one, each time you try to dilate your arteries can occur in as little as one week of practice. More typically, however, it takes several weeks of daily practice to obtain the desired results. This process is considerably speeded up if you use some of the techniques that are discussed in later chapters. The more you practice, the faster you will learn how to control your migraines. Each time you are able to increase your finger temperature, you are gently dilating the arteries supplying blood to your brain making you less vasoconstricted, as well as less susceptible to become vasoconstricted. This means you will be less likely to show an overcorrected vasodilation and a consequent migraine headache.

Some hints that may help

Here are some ideas other people have tried in their biofeedback attempts which may be useful to you. Some people have actually tried to imagine the arteries in their arms, brain, and throughout their bodies opening and allowing more blood and warmth to spread throughout themselves. One person imagined that his arm was hollow and that warm chicken soup was filling up the arm producing a feeling of warmth and well-being. Others have attempted to relax their muscles and hang as loose as possible. (I will have more to say about this muscle relaxation in a later chapter.)

Some of my patients have been successful in increasing their finger temperature when they recalled a memory of a place that was extremely pleasing and comfortable for them. For example, one patient imagined that he was soaking in a pleasant, warm bath. He thought about details like the sounds of the water sloshing around in the tub, the smell of the steam, and the reflections of light off the surface of the water to help recall the situation.

These examples merely illustrate the wide variety of approaches that seem to work for some of my patients. One of my patients told me that he simply did something unnameable which made the spots on the biotic band gradually move up and change color in the increasing-warmth direction. I leave you to your own devices, at least at this point, concerning what you can try to increase your finger temperature. I will give you additional suggestions in a later chapter, but now I would like you to start using the biotic band in the manner that I have suggested. The chances are very good that you will be successful in some of your attempts to raise your finger temperature.

As reassuring as I am, however, this whole procedure might be very frustrating to you because I haven't given you a simple description for how to produce warmth in your hand. "After all," you could say, "it would be easy to ask your patients who were successful handwarmers what it is that they did and then pass this information on to me." Unfortunately, as I have pointed out above, one can only get some hints from these patients. Almost invariably, my patients have a great deal of difficulty in trying to make me understand what it is that they are doing. Even my patients who earn their living from their ability to express themselves (writers, teachers) find themselves at a loss for words when it comes to explaining what they do to voluntarily vasodilate, probably because they never had an opportunity to learn words or labels to describe this new process.

Why say "vasodilate" to yourself?

Earlier in this chapter, I suggested that you say the word "vasodilate" to yourself during your use of the biotic band. There is a definite purpose in saying, "vasodilate," right before each attempt to raise your finger temperature. At this stage, saying this word will probably have no affect on you whatsoever. But as you practice, the word will become a cue that can have considerable power over your arteries, and you can then use this word to your own advantage. This is based on very sound scientific principles; it is not magical or mystical.

You have, I am sure, heard of Dr. Pavlov's famous experiments on dogs that were performed in 1918. Pavlov wanted to find out if he could make his dogs salivate at the mere sound of a bell. He began this experiment by sounding a bell and then checking to see if the dog salivated. As you might guess, at this stage the bell had no effect whatsoever on the dog.

Pavlov then proceeded to "condition" his subject. He did this by first sounding the bell and then, a few seconds later, putting a small amount of food in the dog's mouth. He did this again and again; first the bell, then the food. Gradually, the dog started to respond to the bell as a cue. He began to salivate when the bell was sounded alone—without the food. The relevance of this experiment to you is that salivation is a glandular process that has many similarities to the process of vasoconstriction and vasodilation. In fact, several conditioning experiments on human volunteers have shown that cues can bring about changes in the artery system.

In one such experiment, human volunteers were asked to sit in a comfortable laboratory chair and have attached to their fingers a device called a *plethysmograph,* which directly measures the opening and closing of the arteries in their fingers. In addition to the plethysmograph, a set of wires was attached to the subject which delivered a mild electric shock. The shock was not painful but was noticeable enough so that it automatically produced a vasoconstriction in the arteries in the hand (and, of course, in the head). The experiment proceeded as follows:

Every twenty seconds a word was read over a loudspeaker system so that the subject could hear it. Many different words were presented. For example, "table," "plant," "chair," "pencil," "automobile," "barn." There was no way that the subject could predict on each trial which word he would hear. The mild electric shock was delivered to the subject only after the word "barn" was read over the loudspeaker system. The experiment continued in this manner, i.e., word after word would be spoken and after the word "barn" the shock would occur. The experimenters then turned off the shock apparatus and tried several test words. Each time the word "barn" was presented, the subject showed a vasoconstriction in the fingers even though there was no electric shock.

Vasoconstriction in the fingers did not occur when other words were presented. Whether we like it or not, conditioning is an automatic process that occurs in all people. Just as conditioning was used to make the word "barn" bring about a vasoconstriction, it can also be used to make the word "vasodilate" bring about a vasodilation. By saying the word "vasodilate" to yourself immediately before you actually vasodilate your arteries, you are going to make good use of the conditioning process that will directly benefit you.

The procedures described in this book are designed for you to condition yourself. For example, I asked you to say the cue word to yourself and then try to make your arteries open up through biofeedback. Gradually this sequence will make "vasodilate" a cue word that can automatically bring about an actual vasodilation. The success of this conditioning depends on regular practice of the techniques given in this book.

Difference between warming hands by biofeedback and placing your hand in a pail of warm water

I have often been asked, "Why go through all the trouble of biofeedback training when I can easily warm my hands by placing them in a bowl of warm water." There is a vast difference between warming your hands by opening up the arteries that lead to them and placing your hands in warm water. As you may recall, we are really only interested in your learning how to warm you hands because when you do this, it automatically results in the vasodilation of the arteries in your head.

Placing hands in warm water produces a local response. That is, the warm water will probably affect the arteries in the hand in the water and not necessarily have a marked effect on arteries elsewhere in the body. To the best of my knowledge, nobody has ever avoided a headache by producing a local change in the arteries of the hands. Headaches and the avoidance of headaches come only from changes in the arteries that supply blood to the brain. Through the techniques given in this book, you will be learning a general response for the arteries of your body.

Can biofeedback be harmful?

Biofeedback is generally accepted as a safe and gentle treatment of those disorders for which control over bodily processes is beneficial. There is, however, one possible negative effect of biofeedback: Apparently, for an extremely small percentage of people, any type of relaxation-based treatment (which includes biofeedback, relaxation exercises, meditation) can produce the negative effect of increasing blood pressure.

I would like to emphasize that there has not been any major scientific evidence to show that this negative outcome does occur. But because that possibility does exist, I suggest the following precaution: As you know this book is intended for individuals who are under their doctor's care for headaches. If your doctor does not routinely take your blood pressure, you could ask him/her to do so before you begin the exercises outlined in these pages. If he regularly has taken your blood pressure, then you know what your blood pressure was before you began the techniques given in this book. After you've used the procedures outlined in this book for a week or two, I would recommend that you visit your doctor again and have him check your blood pressure.

I have routinely checked the blood pressure of the many patients I have seen at my clinic. I have yet to find an instance in

Biofeedback procedures tend to reduce blood pressure.

which blood pressure has increased. In fact, I tend to find that bio-feedback procedures tend to reduce blood pressure. In fact, biofeed-back is sometimes used as part of a treatment program for patients who are suffering from high blood pressure.

I emphasize this because I do not want you to overreact to the warning that I have given you. In any event, you certainly can put anxieties and fears to rest by having your blood pressure checked in the manner that I have suggested. It is a good policy, just for general health considerations.

I have only one other piece of advice concerning possible nega-tive effects of biofeedback. If you try the procedures as I have sug-gested and find the experience unpleasant, then the program should be discontinued. The unpleasantness might be experienced as an in-crease in anxiety or tension or a strong emotional reaction that occurs during or immediately after you have completed one of the exercises specified in this book. This does not mean that the approach in this book is not appropriate for you, but it does mean that if you wish to continue, you probably should seek professional help. For a wide variety of reasons, some people have great difficulty in attempting to do relaxation-based procedures. If you happen to be one of these individuals, then I would stop doing whatever makes you feel uncom-fortable. If the procedures that I have suggested are the correct ones for you, they will be experienced as relaxing and comfortable.

What to do if your biotic band reads less than 78 degrees

As I mentioned, it is not unusual for a migraine sufferer to show a temperature of less than 78 degrees. There is, therefore, nothing to be alarmed about if you happen to be one of those individuals. The fact that your reading is below 78 degrees does have some implica-tions on how you are going to use your biotic band: Let us suppose your actual temperature is 68 degrees. This means that when you put on your biotic band none of the squares will be illuminated. The only information that you have at this point is that your temperature is below 78 degrees. There is no way that the biotic band can tell you what your actual temperature is.

Let us now assume that you have followed the instructions giv-en earlier in the chapter. You take your initial reading, and all you know is that it is below 78 degrees. You then begin your attempt at vasodilation by saying the word "vasodilate" to yourself and trying whatever you think may result in an actual vasodilation. You try this for three or four minutes and then open your eyes and look at the biotic band in order to find out what has happened. If one of the dots is now illuminated, you know that you have vasodilated. Even though you can't be sure how much you have vasodilated, the biotic band is giving you the necessary information that is critical for bio-feedback devices to do their job.

However, it may still show no dots illuminated. Therefore, you know only that your temperature is still below 78 degrees. You may in fact, have raised your finger temperature by several degrees, but since the biotic band does not read within your temperature range, you have no way of knowing this. Begin the exercises in chapter 3 at this point anyway and continue to use your biotic band as a temperature indicator. Rather than giving feedback for small changes in temperature, your biotic band will only be able to tell you when your hand temperature has reached the 78 degree level.

Once you pass 78 degrees, you can use the band as a more precise biofeedback device. One consolation: If your hands are quite cool and register below the 78 degree mark, this usually means that you are an especially good candidate for treating migraines in the manner outlined in this book. Further, since your hand temperature is so low, it is likely you can experience a larger change than individuals who already have higher hand temperatures.

How long do you have to keep doing the biofeedback exercises?

As you practice, you will notice that your dependence on the biotic band is gradually reduced until you will no longer need it. Similarly, the relaxation exercises described in the next chapter are initially to be used on a regularly prescribed basis. However, with time you can pattern your own use of these exercises for your maximum benefit.

The migraine headaches that you have are there because of life-long habits combined with your particular physical makeup. As you use the techniques in this book, you will find that your lifelong habits will change into slightly different habits.

The techniques I ask you to practice at this time seem like a purposeful, at times inconvenient, endeavor on your part. Later these techniques will be incorporated into your daily pattern of living. Just as brushing one's teeth or putting on socks is often done automatically, without thought, so will the techniques that prevent you from vasoconstricting become part of your daily life. When this happens, they will no longer be seen as an inconvenience or a nuisance. The benefits of avoiding or reducing migraine headaches are so great that these relatively minor intrusions are hardly even noticed.

The techniques that keep you from vasoconstricting become part of your daily life.

Now that you have read this far—

Up to this point, if you are following my suggestions you are: Trying at least three or four times throughout the day to raise your temperature within a three- or four-minute period using the biotic band for feedback.

3

THE MEDLAX

We're now ready to begin a separate set of exercises designed to help you accomplish even more in your biofeedback attempts. The purpose of practicing these exercises, called the Medlax, is to enhance your ability to raise the temperature of your hands at will and thus prevent or stop vasoconstrictions in your head. Again, there are no shortcuts. Follow precisely the step-by-step instructions that are given to you in this chapter.

In the actual practice or use of the techniques described here, the amount of time involved is really quite small. In addition to the three- or four-minute biofeedback attempts that you are trying several times a day, I ask you to do a very brief, two-minute exercise, the Medlax, every other hour during your waking day. Each time you do the Medlax, and each time you experience the feelings that are associated with it, you are giving the stimulus word "vasodilate" a little extra power to bring about the vasodilation that will help you avoid headaches.

There is a common thread that ties together and integrates the results of your practicing the Medlax and your separate practice sessions using biofeedback. First, both of these techniques are designed to help you bring about vasodilation of the arteries in your head. Second, the word "vasodilate" is an integral part of the Medlax exercise just as it is an integral part of your biofeedback attempts. Through the process of classical conditioning, the benefits of both the Medlax and the biofeedback attempts will be automatically transferred from one to the other. Something akin to a snowballing effect will take place, where the benefit you receive will be more than twice the effect of practicing either one of these techniques alone.

It will take about thirty minutes to learn how to do the Medlax. Once you have mastered the technique by going through this initial thirty-minute experience, thereafter it only takes about two minutes to do the entire exercise. The briefness of the Medlax is a very important feature. Because it is so brief, it means that you can practice it regularly every day without having it interfere with your normal activities.

Practicing the Medlax is quite different from practicing your biofeedback attempts. There is a precise procedure for practicing Medlax with each step carefully spelled out. The detailed procedure for doing Medlax is in sharp contrast to the experimental approach I asked you to follow while trying the three- to four-minute biofeedback attempts. After you have learned the Medlax, you may wish to use part or all of it while you try to warm your hands.

Before describing the exercises themselves, I want to give you the reasons for doing this particular procedure in the way I ask. As with everything in this book, there are precise reasons for what I ask you to do. The brief Medlax exercise is based on two very interesting research topics. The first concerns how muscles that are under your voluntary control can influence and affect your blood vessel system. The second concerns an American scientific inquiry into the eastern technique of meditation.

How muscle tension can produce vasoconstriction

Once again, we must look at the construction of your body and its nervous system so that you can gain an understanding of your migraines. As you know, the brain is the central switchboard which controls and operates a great many of the functions of our body. This highly complex switchboard includes nerves that carry signals to the muscles or organs under its control. In addition, there are nerves which carry impulses from our awareness of the environment, as well as our awareness of our body itself. To make things even more complicated, there are many interconnections *within* the brain, linking together various bodily systems, memory circuits, etc.

Some people are considered to be tense individuals. That is, there is a certain amount of tenseness in the muscles, either throughout or at least in particular regions of the body. Muscles do not remain tense unless there are nervous impulses from the brain directing them to contract. This means that there is a certain amount of continuous nervous impulse activity running down the nerves from the brain to the tensed muscles. Thus, if we were to consider the nervous system of two individuals, one who is somewhat muscularly tense most of the time and the other who is not, we would find one relatively quiet nervous system and another rather active nervous system.

The interesting thing about muscle tenseness is that you may not be aware that you have a certain amount of tension all the time. I have seen many patients who outwardly appear quite relaxed and

You may not be aware that you have a certain amount of tension all the time.

who describe themselves as "laid back" or "very relaxed" but who (I have found through the use of electronic measurement devices) have a certain amount of tenseness all the time.

A very interesting question now arises: Why would you or anybody else have tense muscles for no apparent reason? For example, you are simply sitting down in a chair and resting, you need practically no muscle tension to do this job, yet you maintain a small amount of rigidity or tenseness in your muscular system. In order to answer this question, we again have to go back to the tiger who suddenly jumps out at you and produces automatic reactions in your body. It certainly makes sense for you to tense muscles under such conditions, since maintaining a relaxed muscle state is certainly not going to do any good whatsoever in dealing with the tiger.

According to our theory, although we confront no tigers in our daily lives, we tend to react to the everyday stresses and problems in a manner similar to the way we would react to a real physical threat. Just as you may constrict blood vessels in your head from encountering day-to-day living experiences, you similarly might tense your muscles.

Just as you may constrict blood vessels in your head from encountering day-to-day living experiences, you similarly might tense your muscles.

This is a truly disfunctional or harmful way for you to react—since tense muscles are not going to help you deal with the policeman who is writing out your speeding ticket or your boss who is asking you some questions about your work performance. To make matters even worse, you may hold onto this muscle tension even after the ticket-writing policeman is out of sight or you're no longer in your boss's office. This lingering muscle tension can be seen as an automatic response of our bodies which would be so right and appropriate for dealing with the tiger but is so inappropriate for dealing with the kinds of situations we encounter today.

How muscle tension affects or brings about migraines

Let's go back to considering your brain once again. If you carry around with you a certain amount of unnecessary muscle tension for most of the day, this means the nerves leading from your brain down to the muscles that are tense are relatively active, sending impulses on a regular basis in order to maintain and keep the tension going.

The nerve from the brain to the muscle is a very interesting structure. It is very much like a long wire which starts near the top of your brain and runs all the way down through the lower part of the brain, most likely into the spinal column, finally ending in the muscle itself. At the point, however, where the nerve passes through or near the base of your skull, it branches into two. The main path continues down to the muscle itself, but the little side branch is connected to the brain stem near the base of your skull. This means that the nervous impulse that started out in your brain headed down the nerve to the muscle and also ended up in the brain stem. It is this nervous impulse going into the brain stem that is so terribly important to the victim of migraine headaches.

The brain stem is like a master control unit of the whole nervous system. It determines how much nervous system activity is going on, how awake, drowsy, or alert you might be. It is somewhat like a variable dimmer light switch which controls the lights in a room. When turned on full force, the intensity of the lights can actually hurt your eyes and make it difficult to work.

The more nervous impulses that go into the brain stem, the more it cranks up the overall activity of your nervous system. Thus, the more muscle tension you have, the more you are telling your brain stem to get *all* of your bodily systems into a higher pitch of activity. For the migraine sufferer, this spells trouble because you already have a real problem with an overreactive blood vessel system in your head. The command from your brain stem to increase this activity even more makes you that much more susceptible to vasoconstrictions and the eventual pain of migraines.

I perform a test in my office that is aimed at diagnosing the nature of bodily reactions in migraine sufferers. This consists of accurately measuring muscle tension levels through the use of sophisticated electronic equipment while keeping careful track of hand warmth. After the patient has been connected to the diagnostic instruments, I ask them to rest as best they can for five minutes. By looking at the measurements of temperature and muscle activity, I can find out whether the person tends to be vasoconstricted and/or muscularly tense even though they are trying to relax. Migraine sufferers tend to show a certain amount of coolness in their hands indicating the presence of the vasoconstriction response. The vast majority also show a certain amount of unnecessary muscle activity while they are attempting to relax.

After the rest period, I ask the patient to start with the number 1,000 and successively subtract 7 from it as rapidly as he or she can. At the end of five minutes, I ask for the residual number the patient has calculated, and I tell the patient if it is correct. Patients do this without the aid of pencil and paper or hand calculators. If they get mixed up or think they have made a mistake, they are told to start over again. Ready? Start! As the patient calculates, I carefully look at what happens to their muscles and hand temperature.

Sure enough, muscle tension increases. Sometimes muscles tense throughout the body, but often just in one particular place like the shoulder on the right side or the jaw. At the same time, hand temperature drops even further. How counterproductive my patients tend to be! They do not need muscles to do a mental arithmetic task; they don't need to cut down the amount of blood going into their brain.

To make matters worse, when they have completed the mental arithmetic task, I tell them that it was simply a diagnostic test and that they should forget about it, it's really not important, and try to relax as best they can. Nearly always, they are unable to get their muscle tension level down to its somewhat elevated level at the beginning of the test. And, you guessed it, their arteries remain constricted. Even in the artificial and clinical environment of my office, the migraine sufferer's body reacts to stress as though it has just seen a tiger.

The scientist and the yogi

No one is more skeptical, stern-faced, hard-headed, suspicious, and condescending than the American scientist. He or she basically believes nothing until it has been proven. And even after it has been proven, the scientist still questions whether it is *really* that way or whether some mistake was made in gathering information.

Scientists spend many years learning how to be very critical of grandiose claims. They need evidence, even for the most obvious truths that the layman will accept. For this reason I am always struck with disbelief when I attend a biofeedback convention and see lab-coated scientists mingling and talking to turban-wearing yogis. Remarkable advances in electronic instrumentation and the discovery of biofeedback have brought these two unlikely bedfellows together.

For many, many years, the yogis have claimed that they could control internal bodily processes by various types of mental activity. For many years the scientists scoffed at such claims and focused their attention on the effects of drugs and other strong stimuli on those same bodily processes. Then, a number of experiments done on yogis and Zen masters in India and Japan demonstrated that they can, in fact, do what they have claimed to do for all of these centuries. Once mental activity could be measured, it became respectable for the scientist to look at the mental activities of the yogi and do experiments in order to discover how and why those activities affected the body in the way they did.

At first experimenters took the various yogic and Zen exercises and had ordinary people practice them verbatim, while measurements were taken of blood flow, heart rate, metabolism, brain waves, etc. The effects were remarkable and profound. The question, however, was, did you have to go through and believe all of the things that the eastern mystics believed in order to produce these changes?

After several years of careful experiments, the answer clearly is that you do not have to adopt the eastern mystic's philosophy or way of life in order to produce the physiologic changes that are so beneficial.

In a book called *The Relaxation Response*, Dr. Herbert Benson carefully studied eastern meditation and then stripped away much

You do not have to adopt the eastern mystic's philosophy or way of life in order to produce the physiological changes that are so beneficial.

of the hocus-pocus to get down to the bare essentials needed for it to be effective. The basic essentials are:

1. A word or phrase which is repeated over and over again in the mind of the meditator (this is called the "mantra" by the mystic).

2. A passive attitude maintained by the meditator. This simply means that you cannot try to make anything happen. You simply follow the instructions for meditation, do as the instructions tell you to do, and then let whatever happens, happen. If you find yourself saying things like "I'm not doing it right, it's not working well enough, I should feel more relaxed," then you are not maintaining a passive attitude. It is critical that you allow whatever happens to happen, which includes forgetting to say the mantra.

3. Attention focused on your breathing.

4. The acceptance of extraneous thoughts. It's perfectly okay during meditation to have extraneous thoughts. Once you notice that you have an extraneous thought or are not doing as the instructions have specified, then you gently and easily return to following the exercise as instructed.

Medlax—A meditation-muscle relaxation technique

By carefully following the instructions of this combination technique, you can expect to:

1. Increase your ability to perform the biofeedback exercise.

2. Reduce muscle tension levels and thereby cut down on brain stem activation and overall nervous system activity.

3. Receive the benefits of meditation.

In order to learn how to do the Medlax, find a quiet place with a comfortable chair where you can be alone for about thirty minutes. Once you have gone through this initial thirty-minute training period, you will then be ready to use the three-minute Medlax on a regular basis. If you do not practice the Medlax regularly after you have learned how to do it, you might find it useful to return to the initial thirty-minute training period to refresh your memory of the proper procedures. Some of my patients have also reported that even after they have regularly practiced the Medlax, they like to reread the initial training procedure every few days in order to reassure themselves that they are doing it correctly.

During the next thirty minutes, you will learn to become aware of the six major muscle groups in your body. Learning how to do the Medlax is broken down into eight separate steps, each of which takes about three minutes to complete. Once you have completed these steps in the initial thirty-minute learning phase, you will be ready to start using the three-minute Medlax throughout the day.

To learn the Medlax you should be seated in a chair with both feet flat on the ground and slightly extended in front of the chair. Read through the complete set of instructions for each step before attempting to do the exercise. After you have completed each step, proceed to the next. If you feel any pain or discomfort when your muscles are tensed, eliminate that portion of the exercise.

Step One is the three-minute Medlax exercise as you will be practicing it once you have completed all of the major steps. The first time that you try Step One, you will receive some benefit. When you then return to Step One after proceeding through the additional steps, you will find that your ability to relax by doing the Medlax exercise will be greatly enhanced. Remember, this is the actual Medlax exercise that I ask you to practice every other hour during your waking day.

In order to get the maximum benefit out of doing the Medlax exercise as explained in Step One, it is important to go through the practice exercise in Steps Two through Eight at least one time. Make sure that you take a brief rest between each of the steps, and remember if you have any uncomfortable feelings or begin to feel faint, either discontinue the entire exercise or that portion that produces the discomfort.

Step One—the Medlax

Take a deep breath and hold it. At the same time, tense all the muscles in your body. While you are holding your breath and tensing your muscles for about five seconds, try to notice the location of the muscle tension and the feelings in your tight muscles. After about five seconds, release all of the muscle tension, that is, let your muscles go loose. At the same time, exhale naturally and say the word "vasodilate" to yourself. Allow yourself to breathe naturally about five to ten times and with each expelled breath say the word "vasodilate" to yourself.

Many of my patients like to do this exercise with their eyes closed, although there is no reason why you could not leave your eyes open. Do whatever is most comfortable for you.

As simple as this exercise seems, it has been carefully designed to contain the essential elements of many approaches to using the mind to affect your bodily processes.

Repeat Step One before proceeding to Step Two.

Step Two

In this and the following steps we emphasize different aspects of what you did during Step One. The purpose of this emphasis is to focus your attention on various aspects of the relaxation-meditation process.

During Step Two, proceed exactly as in Step One except do "abdominal breathing" when you take in your initial deep breath and when you do the five to ten naturally occurring breaths thereafter.

To do abdominal breathing, make sure that your stomach moves in and out as you take in and let out air. Try to imagine as you take in the breath that it goes deep into your belly and abdominal area, making those areas extend outward.

To begin Step Two:

1. Take a deep breath, trying to use abdominal breathing, and hold it.
2. Tense all the muscles in your body and hold them tense for about five seconds.
3. Release all muscle tension.
4. Exhale naturally, letting your belly and abdominal areas move inward.
5. While you are relaxing and exhaling, say "vasodilate" to yourself.
6. Allow yourself to breathe naturally, using abdominal breathing, and say "vasodilate" to yourself each time you exhale.
7. Repeat Steps One through Six once more.

Step Three

Proceed exactly as before, using abdominal breathing, except when you take in your deep breath and tighten all your muscles, pay particular attention to the muscles in your legs, your feet, and your thighs. While you are holding your breath, give particular attention to the feelings that are present in those muscles when they are tight. Try pushing the front part of your foot down into the ground while tightening the muscles in your thighs.

At the end of five seconds, exhale, allowing all the muscles in your body to relax, but giving particular attention to the legs, feet, and thighs. At the same time that your muscles are relaxing and your breath is being released, say the word "vasodilate" to yourself. Then, breathing naturally with abdominal movements, say the word "vasodilate" each time you breathe out. As before, continue for about five to ten breaths. Repeat Step Three one more time.

Step Four

As in Steps Two and Three, take a deep breath, using abdominal breathing, and tighten all the muscles in your body, but this time give particular attention to your stomach muscles and your lower back muscles. Make sure these muscles are tensed as best you can, and try to attend to the feelings generated by their tenseness. Again, after five seconds, exhale, release all the tension in your muscles and say "vasodilate" to yourself. Repeat Step Four.

Step Five

Step Five follows the Step Three and Four procedures except that you focus particular attention on the feeling of the tight muscles in your chest and in your upper and lower arms. Because you are holding your breath, your chest will be tense, but you may have to put a little extra effort into tensing your arms to make sure that they are tight also. Repeat Step Five and proceed.

Step Six

This time, when you inhale and tense all the muscles in your body, pay particular attention to your neck and shoulders. You may wish to move your neck to the far right, to the far left, and back and forth to make sure you can experience feelings of tenseness in this area. Shoulder tenseness can also be increased by hunching up the shoulder muscles. After five seconds, release your breath, allow all the muscles in your body to relax, say the word "vasodilate" to yourself and proceed as in previous steps.

Step Seven

During Step Seven, pay particular attention to the muscles in your face, jaw, and forehead. After you have taken your deep breath (remember the abdominal breathing), the tension in these muscles can be sensed better if you are clenching your teeth, wrinkling your forehead, and furrowing your brow.

Again, at the end of five seconds release your breath and release all the muscle tension everywhere in your body, paying particular attention to the facial muscles. You can aid the release of facial muscle tension by relaxing your jaw, allowing your forehead to smooth out, and making a slight smile. While releasing, say "vasodilate" to yourself. Continue to say "vasodilate" each time you breathe out for about the next five to ten breaths. As before, repeat the whole process one more time.

Step Eight

Tighten all the muscles using the awareness you have gained in the previous steps as you take a deep breath. This time focus particular attention on your eye muscles. You can experience the tension in these muscles by moving them to the far right and then to the far left while your eyes are closed. When you relax, you will notice the absence of tension in these muscles completely. Now exhale, release tension in your muscles, and say "vasodilate" to yourself. Again, saying "vasodilate" each time you breathe out for five to ten breaths, repeat the whole process one more time.

After you have completed Step Eight, you are ready to use the Medlax every other hour during the day.

The Medlax exercise is actually Step One by itself. Since you have gone through all eight steps, each time you use the Medlax, you are now aware of various muscle groups and abdominal breathing when you perform the Medlax exercise. Let me repeat:—*In order to do the Medlax, all you do is the Step One procedure.* It is not necessary to repeat all eight steps. (Review is useful if you care to refresh your memory, or if you have not practiced the Medlax for several days and would like a reminder about the various muscle groups and how to do abdominal breathing.)

Now that you have read this far—

You should now be performing two separate exercises during the day:

1. While wearing the biotic band, continue to experiment at least three or four times each day in raising your finger temperature in a three- to four-minute practice period. Reading temperature changes on the biotic band will allow you to assess how well you are doing.
2. Separate from the biofeedback experiments using the biotic band, do the Medlax every other hour during your waking day. Although at first this might seem like a nuisance, it is a very brief exercise and the benefits that can accrue far outweigh the time needed to perform it.

You may use parts or all of this exercise in doing the biofeedback experiments involving the biotic band as suggested above. The choice is yours, and hopefully you will continue to try new and different techniques for raising finger temperature until you are comfortable and confident with the method that you are using.

4

INCREASING YOUR AWARENESS

By this time you are well on your way to learning how to control the arteries in your head, to vasodilate them at will and to stop the onset of migraine headaches. In fact, you already know enough to bring about, in time, pervasive changes in yourself so that you can significantly affect and reduce the suffering from your headaches. There are several little tricks, however, that can greatly speed you along the way in your self-treatment program. This, and the following chapters, will allow you to benefit from the experience of others who had to learn through a trial-and-error method.

You are now using your biofeedback device to teach yourself how to dilate arteries. In time, you will be able to accurately judge the temperature of your hand *without* looking at the biotic band. That is, through the regular use of the biofeedback exercises, you can become aware of your hand temperature by using the sensory systems already present in your body.

The advantages of this newfound awareness are profound. Just from the standpoint of convenience alone, awareness of hand temperature is a worthwhile skill to acquire. First, if you become sensitive enough, you will not have to bother with the biotic band every time you wish to practice your vasodilation skills. This means it will be easier for you to practice hand warming since it can be done anywhere, even if you have forgotten your biotic band. Some of my patients were somewhat embarrassed, although there really is no logical reason to be, to use the biotic band at a social gathering or a busy lunch counter. Learning to become aware of hand warmth without the band can certainly avoid this embarrassment and make it extremely convenient to practice whenever you have a few minutes to spare. Awareness, then, is a convenient and practical skill that will greatly assist you in the coming years.

Like any other skill, awareness can be learned. The process I ask you to learn to become aware is extremely simple. Each time you practice your biofeedback skills (which hopefully you are doing at least three to four times each day), guess what your finger temperature is before you take the initial, or "before," reading on your biotic band. Write this guess down, then read the biotic band to see what your actual fingertip temperature is. By following this simple procedure, you are giving yourself immediate feedback as to how aware or accurate your guess is.

After you have completed your three- to four-minute vasodilation experiment, guess what your fingertip temperature is before reading the "after" temperature. Again, you will get immediate feedback on the accuracy of your guess. If you make these guesses about your temperature before reading the actual temperature each time you do your biofeedback vasodilation experiment, you are then also giving yourself two separate feedback experiences on your awareness skills.

At first, you probably will not be able to accurately guess what your temperature is. As with learning any new skill, it takes persistence and practice before you become proficient. As I have stressed previously, it is important for you to write down your guesses and actual temperature readings during your vasodilation attempts. In this manner, you can refer back to previous experiences to see what your progress is. You are not going to become an excellent "vasodilator" or "finger-warmth awareness guesser" overnight. But, with practice, you will be amazed at how tuned-in you can become to your own bodily functions.

Let's review at this point what you are doing to help yourself get over your migraine headaches. First, three to four times each day, you are using biofeedback to help you learn vasodilation skills while wearing the biotic band. Second, during each of these biofeedback practice sessions, you are making *two guesses* of your fingertip temperature before you read the actual temperature on the biotic band. Third, you are practicing the Medlax every other hour during the day.

Although this sounds like a lot, it amounts to only a few minutes a day. Eventually, you will find your own pattern and spacing of these various exercises so that they will become second nature and as much a part of your life as sleeping and eating. Best of all, of course, is that the few minutes spent on a daily basis can save untold hours and days of pain and lost time from your overreactive artery system and consequent migraines.

Warning

Becoming aware seems like a simple convenience to aid you with your vasodilation exercises. I must warn you, however, that something else might happen once you become aware of your hand temperature without using the biotic band. I gave you this warning not because there are any dangers involved but because you may

You may learn something about yourself that you have not wanted to face before.

learn something about yourself that you have not wanted to face before. Perhaps that's a little too strong. I don't really think you will learn anything totally new about yourself. Instead you may discover something that you know at some level of awareness but have not really reckoned with completely. To illustrate how awareness of hand temperature can lead to knowledge about yourself, let's refer back to the caveperson ten thousand years ago, who is happily walking down a path and hears a growl from behind some bushes.

If this caveperson had, as you have been doing, used a biofeedback device to become aware of hand temperature, he would have noticed that a drop or vasoconstriction occurred immediately after the growl. He then could have said to himself, "Isn't that amazing? A growl from behind the bushes made me vasoconstrict. My body truly is reacting to that growl as though it were a threat. If I'm going to avoid vasoconstrictions, I'm going to have to avoid such threatening occurrences in the future. Perhaps I'll just stay in my cave, or maybe I won't take this particular path anymore."

Just as our caveperson is now aware that a stimulus in the environment, a growl, can produce a vasoconstriction, you might similarly become aware of danger signals in your environment that make you vasoconstrict. Unlike the growl for the caveperson, however, the danger signals in your environment might puzzle you because in actuality, these events are not life-endangering threats. A call from your mother to find out how you are doing may result in a vasoconstriction, or an interaction with your husband about what to do on the weekend may result in a vasoconstriction. Your new sensitivity, in other words, can lead to an awareness of psychological threats and disturbances in your environment.

> Your new awareness can lead to an awareness of psychological threats and disturbances that are in your environment.

The warning to you is that awareness of vasoconstrictions may result in a very explicit awareness of some things that you preferred not to think about. Although this notion might be somewhat uncomfortable at first, it can really help you since the only way one can ever attempt to solve a problem is to be aware of it in the first place.

Learning how to control your hand temperature and the arteries in your head is going to do a great deal for you in terms of controlling your migraine headaches. The finishing touches, however, are going to require you to do something about those threats that produce the vasoconstriction in the first place. I'm not saying that you have to change your life so that you no longer are confronted by psychologically threatening events. I am saying, however, that it is useful to be aware of what those events are and to do something about those which can be changed. The following chapters will help you deal with those occurrences in your daily life to which you react as though they were a growl in the bushes or a wild tiger suddenly confronting you. I suggest some fairly direct techniques that are not hard to put into practice. The overall goal is to allow you to gain control of your arteries and eliminate your headaches.

Whatever your level of awareness of finger temperature is at the present time, you should make as much use of this as possible. Even a small amount of awareness can now be used to help you prevent or reduce the pain of migraine headaches. If you notice or think that you have vasoconstricted, use whatever skills you have at your disposal to reverse the vasoconstriction. Even if you can increase your finger temperature just a small amount, and you notice or suspect that you have just vasoconstricted, take a moment to say "vasodilate" to yourself and do whatever you think will stop this vasoconstriction.

Basically, I am suggesting that you begin to use your vasodilation skills to reverse or reduce a vasoconstriction once it has occurred. This will help you prevent your headaches. Up to this point, I have suggested that you practice your biofeedback attempts and Medlax on a regular basis whether you feel you are vasoconstricted or not. As you may recall, I likened this to a preventive maintenance approach on your automobile. What I am suggesting to you now is analogous to maintenance on your automobile when you notice that it's not running quite well or when you hear a squeaky sound. In your case, the preventive care is vasodilating your arteries.

Basically I am suggesting that you begin to use your vasodilation skills to reverse or reduce a vasoconstriction once it has occurred. This will help prevent your headaches.

Now that you have read this far—

At this point, you should be doing the following to eliminate or reduce your migraine pain:

1. Using the biotic band to try to raise your finger temperature within a three- to four-minute period, at least three or four times each day. How you accomplish this is up to you; you can incorporate the suggestions I have given, portions or all of the Medlax exercise, or anything else that you think might help you get the most temperature increase in this brief period of time.

2. Guessing what your finger temperature is before you read the biotic band. You can do this each time you begin the biofeedback attempt and each time you finish. This practice of guessing your temperature before actually reading the biotic band will help you become more and more aware of your finger temperature without use of the biotic band.

3. Practicing the Medlax exercise in the manner that I have suggested at least once every other hour during your waking day.

4. Using whatever skills you have to reverse a drop in finger temperature when you notice or even suspect that one has occurred.

5

DANGER SIGNALS

Up to now I have focused on what you can do directly to your internal bodily reactions to prevent migraines. The emphasis has been on the self-control of the arteries to avoid vasoconstriction or to get rid of a vasoconstriction once it has occurred. Since a vasoconstriction is the first step in the sequence of events that lead to a migraine headache, it is important to do something about a vasoconstriction in order to ultimately avoid the migraine headache itself. The use of biofeedback and the other techniques discussed in previous chapters can go a long way toward preventing or stopping vasoconstrictions. It is even possible that some people can stop reading the book at this point since they may have already sufficiently reduced or even eliminated their headaches just by using the techniques given so far. I have found, however, that many of my patients need some additional skills in order to master their migraine pain.

Another way of looking at the headache pain control techniques discussed in this book is to classify them into (1) those used for directly controlling the internal bodily environment (Medlax, biofeedback) and (2) those used for controlling bodily reactions to the external environment. At this point, I want to shift attention to the world in which you live with particular attention to those situations that produce vasoconstrictive reactions in you. As we move through our daily lives, we encounter danger signals in the world that surrounds us. A danger signal is any event in the external environment that triggers a vasoconstrictive response. In the previous chapter I warned you that becoming aware of your hand temperature might lead you to realizing that you react to many daily situations as though they were danger signals. You may have discovered that vasoconstrictions (as indicated by temperature drops in your hand) are triggered by such situations as your children disobeying you, discovering you have overdrawn your bank account, being told by your boss that you made a mistake, not being invited to a social event, being late for an

A danger signal is any event in the external environment that triggers a vasoconstrictive response.

54

appointment, receiving a phone call from your mother, working on a project to meet a deadline, being sexually refused by your spouse, forgetting to take care of a household task, disagreeing with a sales clerk.

The list could go on and on and could include almost any situation concerning making mistakes, rejection by others, fears of doing poorly, dealing with authorities or superiors, family problems, and receiving or giving criticism. Since these events occur almost on a daily basis and since it is important for you to learn how to avoid the vasoconstrictions produced by these situations, we are going to make a careful analysis of why you regard these situations as danger signals and what can be done to change this manner of reacting.

Danger signals and emotional upsets

Before we analyze danger signals and what can be done about them, I want to point out the relationship between danger signals and emotional upsets that you may experience. Any stimulus that produces a vasoconstriction is a danger signal. Often, however, we can also feel emotionally upset when a danger signal has occurred. That is, a danger signal always produces a vasoconstriction, but quite often it is also experienced as an emotional upset. The clearest example of this type of situation is what happens to your arteries and your emotional state when you suddenly notice a speeding car bearing down on you while crossing the street. In addition to the vasoconstriction and drop in temperature in your hands, you experience fear and anxiety. The danger signal has thus produced a physiological change (vasoconstriction), as well as an emotional upset (fear).

As I have pointed out, it is important for you to be aware of vasoconstrictions so that you can then do something to avoid or stop them. I have emphasized becoming aware of temperature drops in your hand in order to become aware of when a vasoconstriction has occurred. You now have another signal or sign that a vasoconstriction has occurred: If you become emotionally upset, i.e., angry, depressed, frustrated, anxious, you can use these emotional feelings as an indication that a vasoconstriction has occurred.

You can use emotional feelings as an indication that a vasoconstriction has occurred.

I understand that emotional upsets are already unpleasant and my telling you that they also set you up for a migraine headache could even make the experience worse. However, I strongly believe that awareness can lead to real solutions to those conditions that produce vasoconstrictions and the emotional upsets. The important thing is to become aware of the state of your arteries. Now you can use emotional upsets to your advantage since they too can give you information about your arteries.

When you become tense, frustrated, angry, or even depressed, you are also becoming vasoconstricted, and you can conclude that a

Many of us have learned to suppress or avoid feeling the unpleasantness associated with emotional upsets by simply not experiencing them.

danger signal has been perceived in your environment. Although emotional reactions are often associated with danger signals, it is not necessary that the emotional response be present. It is, therefore, possible for you to run into a danger signal, experience a vasoconstriction, and not be aware of any emotional upset whatsoever. This occurs because many of us have learned to suppress or avoid feeling the unpleasantness associated with emotional upsets by simply not experiencing them. Your body, however, knows when you have perceived a danger signal and automatically vasoconstricts whether or not you experience an emotional upset.

As you read this chapter on how to avoid danger signals, you are going to receive a side benefit: If you are one of those individuals who also experiences emotional upset when a danger signal has been presented, you will learn how not to become upset as much or as often as you presently do.

Too many danger signals—isn't it SAD?

You probably have the impression that whether a danger signal does or does not occur in your environment, there is very little you can do about it. Nothing can be further from the truth. Ninety-eight percent of the danger signals that you encounter can be avoided. The occurrence of danger signals not only depends on what you happen to run into in the environment but also upon your own analysis of what happens. SAD describes the sequence of events that leads to a danger signal and your role in determining which situations are seen as danger signals and which are not.

The S in SAD stands for *stimulus*. A stimulus is anything in your external environment to which you react. Several possible stimuli have been mentioned—events like a child disobeying you, a poor evaluation from a professor or a deadline for a report. These stimuli *by themselves*, however, are not automatically a danger signal.

The A *(analysis)* in SAD is critical for a stimulus to be a danger signal. Your *analysis* of the stimulus will determine whether or not the stimulus, in fact, constitutes a danger signal. The analysis at times may be so fast that you are not even aware of it. At other times, the analysis may be quite noticeable. You may talk to yourself and tell yourself things about the stimulus that has just occurred.

A, or *analysis*, then, refers to the conscious, and sometimes unconscious, thinking process that you go through each times a stimulus occurs. Any self-talking or self-statements that you make within your own mind are often an analysis of a stimulus that has occurred. The kind of thought processes that go on when trying to fit a word into a crossword puzzle or calculating if there is enough time to do a number of different errands and tasks within the next two hours are good examples of analysis.

Some stimuli happen so fast that it seems as though your reaction occurs without any analysis. In reality, however, you had to *learn* as a child that certain stimuli, like a speeding car, for example, were dangerous. When you see the speeding car coming down at you, you use your previous experience to make that sight a danger signal. Similarly, when a sales clerk is impolite or rude to you and you vasoconstrict, you may or may not be aware of the analysis that you made after the stimulus (rude statement) and before the vasoconstriction occurred. In any event, an analysis based on your previous life experience must take place before nearly any stimulus can serve as a danger signal.

Finally, the *D* in *SAD*. The *D* stands for danger signal. It is the last term in the sequence of events: Stimulus-Analysis-Danger signal (SAD). Whenever you vasoconstrict, it means that a *D* or *danger signal* has been perceived. Similarly, whenever a danger signal is perceived, it was preceded by a stimulus and your analysis of whether or not that particular stimulus was a danger signal. You may not be aware of your analyzing behavior that determines danger signals, but we are going to look closely at this process so that something can be done about vasoconstrictions produced by environmental stimuli. Although you may not be able to change a stimulus that occurs in your environment, it is often possible to change your analysis of the stimulus as a danger signal.

> In any event, an analysis based on your previous life experience must take place before nearly any stimulus can serve as a danger signal.

> Although you may not be able to change a stimulus that occurs in your environment, it is often possible for you to change your analysis of the stimulus that makes it into a danger signal.

What causes danger signals?

You cause most of the danger signals to which you react. Since the only way a danger signal can occur is through Stimulus-Analysis-Danger signal (SAD) and since the whole process of analysis is one that you control, it logically follows that you are responsible for danger signals.

I do not want you to get the impression, however, that all danger signals are to be avoided. Some danger signals are functional and serve a useful and valuable purpose. These functional danger signals can save your life. They can prepare you to avoid an onrushing car, to get away from a combatant enemy or to strike out against and deter an attacking dog.

Other danger signals are not useful and may even get in the way of your living your life as you would like. These *dysfunctional danger signals* can cloud your thinking so that you make poor decisions, say things that you later regret, and unnecessarily cause a migraine headache. In this chapter we are going to look at ways you can avoid dysfunctional danger signals. These signals often cause emotional upsets, as well as set you up for migraine headaches.

Let's apply the SAD system to our fictitious caveperson who roamed the forest several thousand years ago. Try to put yourself in

> You cause most of the danger signals to which you react.

that caveperson's shoes, or bare feet, and imagine you are walking down the forest path. You have just had a good meal of berries and the weather is fine. You feel quite content and have a pleased smile on your face. Suddenly the bushes rustle. Almost instantaneously you freeze in your steps, a coordinated group of physiological changes involving your heart, lungs, muscles, and glandular system takes place. Your pleased and contented feeling is now replaced by one of fear and stress. The arteries feeding blood to your brain quickly constrict. Then, much to your relief, a porcupine steps out from behind the bushes, and once he spots you becomes even more frightened than you were. The sudden drop in tension and stress that you experience may even lead you to laugh and say to yourself, "I don't know why I became so frightened. That silly old porcupine couldn't hurt a flea."

The question I have is: What caused the physiologic reactions in your caveperson's body when the rustle of the branches and leaves first occurred? The stimulus of rustling bushes by itself cannot be a danger signal. We have all heard trees and bushes rustle in parks and wooded areas and probably have not vasoconstricted or reacted to this situation as though it were a danger signal. In fact, many people find the sound pleasant. This is true for almost any given stimulus, i.e., it produces a danger signal reaction in some people and an entirely different reaction in other people.

This makes perfectly good sense when we apply our SAD system to this situation. The *S* is a rustling sound of bushes, the *A* is the caveperson analyzing the situation and determining that a ferocious animal is behind the bushes and ready to leap with a vicious enthusiasm, causing a loss of life or limb. The *D*, of course, is the danger signal which automatically produces in the body a set of reactions, including vasoconstriction of the arteries leading to the head.

If the caveperson had analyzed the situation differently—for example, if he had said to himself, "The rustle in the bushes *might* be a ferocious animal, but on the other hand it might be just the wind or a harmless animal"—then the automatic physiological response would have been considerably smaller. The caveperson would have been alert and would have gone to discover what really was behind those bushes before going into a full-fledged physiological stress reaction. I believe that most of the danger signals you experience can be eliminated or greatly reduced if you take time to analyze the stimulus more completely and objectively.

> I believe that most of the danger signals you experience can be eliminated or greatly reduced if you take time to analyze the stimulus more completely and objectively.

Analysis that leads to danger signals

Let's go over the process by which danger signals are produced once more. Using the SAD system, first a Stimulus occurs, then you Analyze that stimulus and, depending upon that analysis, a *D*anger signal can automatically occur, calling forth appropriate physiological responses.

The analysis that leads to a danger signal requires a little closer look. As pointed out earlier, the analysis may be so rapid so that you are not even aware of it, or it may involve quite a bit of self-talking, figuring, and so on. Every analysis has a conclusion or bottom line. When you go through the process of analysis and have figured, planned or considered everything that you wish to consider, a conclusion is reached. It is something akin to feeding a computer a great deal of information, having it analyze the information and when the analysis is complete, receiving an output or conclusion. When you do your analyses of stimuli, the conclusion is critical in determining whether or not you will react to the stimulus as a danger signal. There are really only two conclusions that should make your body react as though a danger signal were present.

If your analysis leads to the general conclusion that (1) your life or limb are being threatened, or (2) a law of nature has been violated, you will automatically respond by secreting adrenalin, increasing your heart rate, vasoconstricting the arteries in your hands and head and tensing your muscles. Whenever you go through an analysis of a stimulus and you arrive at one of these two conclusions, your body automatically reacts as though a danger signal were presented. Your body reacts in quite a literal fashion and does not question whether or not your analysis was correct or incorrect. Physically, the body awaits only the conclusion or results of your analysis and responds accordingly.

Even though you might not be aware that one or both of these conclusions have been reached through your analysis, whenever your body reacts to a stimulus with a vasoconstriction, and/or you become emotionally upset, one or both of these conclusions have in fact been reached.

Let us now look at an example of how the SAD system was actually applied to a migraine sufferer and her reactions to her husband's criticism.

The vasoconstrictions of Helen C.

Although Helen had had an occasional migraine or two after she reached adolescence and into her early twenties, they had become increasingly frequent over the past seven years. Usually, once or twice a week, her head pain would be so severe that she required an injection of a potent pain killer and a long period of bed rest and sleep before she could continue her active life. In addition to caring for her family of three children, she did a considerable amount of volunteer work helping less-advantaged children. She loved her husband, Henry, very much and felt they had generally a very good relationship.

After going through the initial phases of treatment using biofeedback to reduce and prevent vasoconstrictions, she was able to significantly reduce both the number and severity of her headaches. Rather than getting one or two severe headaches each week, Helen would only get one or two headaches each month, and they tended not to be as severe or debilitating as they had been in the past. The Medlax and biofeedback helped her to greatly reduce the amount of pain and discomfort that she experienced. Atlhough many people would be satisfied at this point, Helen wanted to see if she could reduce her headache pain even more and perhaps eliminate the headaches completely.

Through biofeedback training, she became very aware of her hand and fingertip temperature. She was able, through the use of biofeedback and relaxation skills, to regularly warm her hands as a preventive measure and could stop many vasoconstrictions when they occurred. She noted, however, that whenever she did something "stupid" and her husband was critical of her, her hand temperature would drop considerably and she was usually unable to interrupt vasoconstrictions caused in this way.

After Helen discovered this relationship between vasoconstrictions and her sensitivity to her husband's reactions, she felt that it was probably normal for her to react this way. She thought that it was inevitable for her to feel tense, nervous, and to vasoconstrict when her husband was displeased and critical of her. I assured her, however, that this danger signal was unnecessary and, further, that she was manufacturing it herself through her *analysis* of her husband's response. Helen was probably not even aware that she did this analysis.

By applying our SAD system we find that: The *S* is Henry being critical of Helen. Helen is vasoconstricting and also feeling upset and tense, therefore, a *D* or *danger signal* has occurred. What was Helen's *analysis* that resulted in the danger signal?

We already know the conclusion of Helen's analysis. That is, since a danger signal was produced, we know that Helen's analysis led to the conclusion that (1) the stimulus was a threat to her life or limb, or (2) a law of nature had been violated.

Let's go through what Helen thought as she analyzed the stimulus to arrive at these conclusions. When Henry criticized Helen, she first thought that she *shouldn't* have done the stupid thing and, further, that Henry *should always* think well of her and like her every moment of every day. I would like to point out the use of the word *should* in both of these thoughts that Helen had.

I want to show you how the use of the word *should* in Helen's thinking and analysis led to and produced the danger signal which caused the vasoconstriction. A danger signal will occur whenever you believe that something *should* happen and, in fact, that something does not happen. *Should* is a very strong word.

In the real world there are only a few things that probably should happen. For example, when you take in a breath of air, there *should* be sufficient oxygen so that you will not suffocate. It would certainly be a horrendous event if there were not sufficient oxygen; it also would be a clear-cut threat to your life, and a law of nature would be violated. Similarly, there *should* be sufficient gravity on earth to make sure we do not float up into space, explode, and die. If there were not sufficient gravity as there *should* be, it would be a horrendous and terrible event. We have come to expect oxygen in our air and gravity beneath our feet. The loss of either of these would, no doubt, lead us to an analysis for which we would appropriately have severe physiologic stress reactions.

Notice that these two *should*s, air and gravity, are highly appropriate uses of the word *should* since we always do have oxygen in our air and gravity beneath our feet. It is not appropriate to use the word *should* in the sentence, "I *should* be rich." No matter how clever or hard-working you are, there is no law of nature that says you *should* be rich. However, if you truly believe that you *should* be rich and you are not rich, you can only conclude that a law of nature has been violated. You will automatically produce a danger signal to which you will physiologically react. It is important to keep in mind, however, that a true law of nature has not been violated in this case. It is just that your use of the word *should* in an inappropriate manner has led you to the conclusion that a violation has occurred. In a sense, you have tricked your body.

As I pointed out earlier, your body and its physical reactions do not question your thinking or analysis. You must use your intellect as best you can to make sure your analysis is correct and appropriate. Once you use the word *should* and then confront the situation in which your *should* does not occur, you have concluded *de facto* that a law of nature has been violated. Thus, if you have vasoconstricted and are under a great deal of stress because you are not rich when you think you should be, it would be inappropriate to think that the stimulus, lack of money, was the danger signal. You yourself have caused the danger signal by using the word *should* as if wealth were a law of nature.

Helen's reaction to her husband Henry would have been appropriate if a law of nature had been violated. In fact, the only law that had been violated was one that Helen manufactured in her own mind through the use of the word *should*: "I *should* not do stupid things" and "Henry *should* love me all of the time."

Before discussing what you can do about analysis that causes your body to overreact, I want you to remember that when you see a danger signal and experience emotional upsets, this means that your

A danger signal will occur whenever you believe that something should happen and, in fact, that something does not happen.

analysis has led you to conclude that a law of nature has been violated or there is a threat to life or limb. Once you are aware of a danger signal, it can be used as a cue that it is time to examine and reanalyze what has happened. Was there a true threat to life or limb? Was a law of nature violated? Or did you simply manufacture these conclusions in your own mind?

There are three steps that you would follow in attempting to eliminate an unnecessary danger signal. Keep in mind that you can never be sure a danger signal is necessary or unnecessary until you have reanalyzed your own thinking processes.

1. When you notice you have vasoconstricted and/or are emotionally upset, say to yourself, "A SAD sequence has occurred." Because of your reaction, you know definitely that a danger signal has occurred, so you also know that an S and an A must be present.

2. Next, identify the stimulus in the SAD sequence. What just happened or is happening in the external world? The stimulus can include anything that somebody else does or says to you, as well as your own external behaviors. Examples of the former would be receiving a letter with bad news, hearing a negative comment, looking at your child's report card, noticing the time and seeing that you forgot an appointment. Examples of the latter would be making a mistake, balancing a checkbook and finding out that you are overdrawn, looking at your desk and seeing all of the uncompleted tasks that have to be done. After you have discovered the stimulus, proceed to step 3.

3. This step is the most demanding; it is the reanalysis of the A in SAD. It requires a good deal of talking to yourself. The first question to ask is, What is the threat to life or limb? Remember, we are talking about real threats: a car racing at you, a person threatening you, etc.

In step 3, be on the lookout for the use of the word *should*. Also be on the lookout for a tendency to make the event seem catastrophic, as when one incorrectly concludes that there is a threat to life or limb when there is not. Two examples are: assuming that you have been fatally injured when you receive a small cut or thinking that you will be without food and shelter when you have just been fired from your job. In both of these cases, a careful and thoughtful consideration of the facts would lead you to less catastrophic conclusions.

Another manner by which you can incorrectly conclude that your life or limb has been threatened is through the improper use of the word need. A need refers to what is required to maintain life and health. There are only three needs; food, water and shelter. We do not need a sports car, a spouse's or parent's love, or admiration from others in order to maintain our life and health. As you do your reanalysis, see if you are using the word *need* in relation to the stimulus. If you find you are using *need*, replace it with *I would like* or, *I wish*.

If there has been no actual threat to life or limb (like a speeding car), then you must have concluded in your previous analysis that a law of nature was violated. It is now up to you to determine what law may have been violated. Is it a true law of nature or one that you have manufactured by your own thinking? A key to determining this is to look at the use of the word *should* in your thinking about the stimulus. If you can discover the *should*, you can then decide if *should* is appropriate for the stimulus situation.

If you discover you are using *should* or *always* in inappropriate ways, then replace those words with *I would like it if*, *it would be nice if*, and so on. It is very important to restate your thoughts without the use of the words *should, need, always*, and without making them seem catastrophic. You might, therefore, end up with a statement like, I would like it if Marvin loved me, but he apparently does not, instead of, I need Marvin's love.

When you are through with your reanalysis, it is important to say the following to yourself: "There is no real threat to my life or limb," or "a law of nature has not been violated." Then, to do something about unnecessary danger signals: (1) Say to yourself, "A *S-A-D* has occurred;" (2) Identify the *S;* (3) Discover what your faulty analysis was and reanalyze. When you are through with this reanalysis, state the new conclusions that help you stop the danger signal.

Let's see how this system helped another migraine sufferer.

William and Mary

William was a twenty-six-year old management trainee in banking when he came to see me about his migraine headaches. He had been having migraines since he entered college, but they occurred at what, for him, was a manageable level. Perhaps once or twice during the academic quarter his headaches would become so bad that he was unable to study or function properly. These typically would come after he had completed a paper or an exam and, therefore, did not markedly interfere with his progress through the university.

The headaches seemed to occur more frequently and with more intensity after he graduated and began his work career. At the time of graduation, he also moved in with Mary, his friend of several years' acquaintance. William and Mary had pretty well committed themselves to living together for the rest of their lives. Although they weren't married, William felt that marriage was a relatively minor step compared to the commitments that they had made to each other.

Both his career and his relationship eventually became a source of stress for William. The relationship finally ended when Mary announced that she was going to leave him to pursue her career in a different city. As he describes it, he was broken-hearted and frustrated because no matter what he offered, he could not convince her to stay with him. Further, his career was being affected by the increasingly frequent severe migraine headaches. At the time he came to see me he was very depressed over this whole state of affairs.

As part of William's regular weekly visits to my office, I took temperature readings of his hands during the biofeedback trianing sessions. As you might guess, he showed consistent coolness of the hands, indicating that he was in an almost constantly vasoconstricted state. Most of the therapeutic hours, however, were devoted to trying to unravel the SADs William encountered that resulted in his body receiving the signal to react as though a life-threatening danger were present. Actually William was manufacturing within himself several erroneous threats to life and violations of laws of nature that resulted in his inability to cope both physically and mentally with his current life situation.

William noticed himself becoming more depressed and upset when he got home at night and saw that Mary was no longer there. He would be reminded of her by pieces of furniture and other mementos that they had acquired while together. The *S* in the SAD sequence for William was seeing that Mary was not there. This resulted in a *D* or danger signal.

Let's look at William's analysis: William apparently believed that Mary *should* be the way he wanted her to be. He felt that since he loved and was devoted to his companion, she *should* return his love and be devoted to him. Now, there is no law of nature that says when you are loving, devoted, kind, etc., to another person, they will return these same feelings to you. In fact, as a psychologist who has dealt with many couples having relationship problems, I can tell you that frequently there is not a fair exchange of considerations in a relationship.

After some discussion, William agreed that there was really no law of nature that said his friend had to be the way he wanted her to be. He agreed to replace the sentence, "She should be and do what I want," with, "It would be nice and I would like it if she would be and do what I want." William also said, "There is no threat to life or limb and a law of nature has not been violated."

There is a great difference between the two sentences that William used in his analysis and reanalysis regarding Mary. In the first case, the word *should* is used, and William's statement takes the form of a law of nature. Since Mary did not do what William thought she *should* do, William was giving his body a signal that a law of nature had been violated. His body did not question his analysis, and his arteries appropriately vasoconstricted. When William

replaced the word *should* with *I would like it* or *it would be nice if,*
then he was able to respond to the facts of his life in a more reasonable manner.

After his reanalysis, whenever William noticed that he was reacting with a danger signal to a stimulus that reminded him that
Mary was gone, he would say to himself, "A law of nature is not
being violated. It would be nice if Mary returned my love and remained with me. However, I am not getting what I would like."
Although he was disappointed and unhappy, William no longer gave
his body the signal that a law of nature had been violated.

William put this insight into practice on a daily basis. Whenever he became aware of his thoughts leading to an emotional upset
and danger signal, he would say to himself, "I am behaving as
though a law of nature has been violated. There is no law of nature
that says that she has to do and be what I want. I would prefer it if
she would do what I want. However, people will not always do what
I want, and I do not have to become extremely emotionally upset."
William would repeat these phrases and argue within his own mind
regarding his analysis until he noticed that the physical reaction and
emotional upset tended to disappear or decrease to a manageable
level.

Let's go on to a few more of William's analyses and see how he
reanalyzed and replaced them with more reasonable ones. Because
of all of the emotional upset and stress in this young man's life, he
was not performing well on his job. Each time he made another
mistake or received some negative feedback from a superior, he analyzed these events and concluded that a life-threatening danger was
present. William apparently told himself that if he didn't do well at
his job, he would be a total failure in life. He would not be able to
obtain another job, nor would he ever be happy at any other kind of
work. He also thought that each time he made a mistake or received
some unfavorable feedback from his boss, he would most certainly
lose his job and, therefore, be a worthless and unhappy person for
the rest of his life. William's body responded to these ideas as though
they were correct. That is, his body reacted as though a mistake
meant he was a worthless person doomed to unhappiness and unable
to provide food and shelter for himself.

William again examined his analysis and replaced it with a
more reasonable one: Just as he had used his bodily reactions as a
signal to reanalyze and replace his self-statements in regard to his
relationship, he did the same thing when he made a mistake on his
job or received negative feedback from his superior. When either of
these occurred and he became vasoconstricted and emotionally upset, he said to himself, "I am reacting as though this is a life-threatening event. It is not catastrophic; I must be giving my body the
signal that my life is being threatened. I'm going to think to myself
the following: (1) An error or negative feedback does not mean that

I will lose my job; (2) even if I do lose my job it does not mean I'm worthless as a human being and will be unable to meet my needs."

Again, through diligent practice William was able to reduce the vasoconstriction and emotional upset that occurred after he made mistakes or had a bad interaction with his boss. He also told himself that it was perfectly okay to make mistakes since nobody is perfect and as long as he is a member of the human race that includes him.

William gradually learned how to stop giving his body signals that his life was being threatened. He combined the use of reanalysis of the S in SAD with biofeedback training to make sure that his body was in a relaxed state as much as possible and that as few vasoconstrictions occurred as was possible.

A number of things happened. First, his depression began to lift and he started to feel better about himself and the things he was doing. Second, his migraine headaches went away, and since he was no longer vasoconstricting as much and starving his brain for blood it needed to function properly, his performance on his job actually began to improve. The last I heard, he was being considered for a major promotion.

I gave you the example of William to illustrate the steps that are necessary to prevent SADs or to reduce their impact and protect yourself from those vasoconstrictions that could lead to the severe pain of a migraine.

You can begin taking these steps the moment that you are aware that a vasoconstriction has occurred or that you are emotionally upset:

1. Say to yourself, "A SAD has occurred, and I'm giving my body a signal that a life-threatening event has occurred or that a law of nature has been violated."

2. Identify the S in SAD.

3. Carefully examine your thoughts and discover how you analyzed the S that led to the faulty conclusion regarding a life-threatening event or violation of nature. You can use certain clues to help you discover what this faulty analysis consisted of. The clues include the use of the words *should, need* and *catastrophic*, or *seeing unreasonable consequences*. Next, vigorously question your analysis within your own mind and perform a reanalysis that seems more reasonable and fitting to the occasion. Once you have reanalyzed, make the new statements to yourself again and again until you can feel the emotional upset completely disappear or greatly diminish.

My patients have often told me that, even though this system seems to work, they are usually not aware of their unreasonable analyses within themselves. They do not actually hear themselves espousing these beliefs when the emotionally upsetting events occur. Admittedly, their bodies react as though these unreasonable beliefs are present, but my patients are not consciously aware of them. Typically the analyses that tend to get us into trouble are so ingrained and part of the fabric of our personality that we no longer have to say them to ourselves consciously to experience the effects of these dysfunctional thoughts.

To discover these faulty analyses, we must act as psychological detectives working backward from the reaction of our body and deducing logically what our analysis must have been. The proof of the pudding, of course, occurs when we reanalyze and arrive at a new, reasonable analysis, start restating it to ourselves and notice that our emotional and physical reactions are affected.

Being a SAD detective

I am asking you to eliminate SADs by reanalyzing your thought processes that produce the danger signals. As I mentioned previously, many of my patients are not aware that they essentially are saying to themselves, "A law of nature has been violated."

Very few people would ever use the exact words *law of nature*. When they do their analysis of the stimulus that has occurred, there may not be any words whatsoever that the patient is aware of. We do know, however, that the analysis does occur and, in one way or the other, does lead to the aforementioned conclusion. We know this occurs because we have deduced, much in the manner that a detective deduces, what must happen to produce the automatic physiological responses in your body. For you to be effective in your battle against vasoconstrictions, it would be desirable for you to also act as a detective who uses clues to determine the truth.

Every detective starts out with evidence that a crime has been committed. It is then a process of working backward to fill in the facts and find the culprit. There are several bits of evidence that you can look at to discover if, in fact, the crime of vasoconstriction has been committed. First, if you had on your biotic band and also happened to notice that there was a rapid temperature drop, let's say several degrees in less than a minute, then you can conclude that a vasoconstriction occurred. Even if you didn't have your biotic band on at the time, you may now be aware of your fingertip temperature through your biofeedback practice sessions. You simply might have noticed that there was a cooling down of the temperature of your fingers; again, evidence that a vasoconstriction has occurred.

Finally, you may not have had your biotic band on or learned how to be aware of fingertip temperature, but you might have noticed that you became emotionally upset. This emotional upset is pretty good evidence that a vasoconstriction occurred. So, now that you know a vasoconstriction occurred, you begin to work backward using new knowledge about your body and danger signals in order to root out the culprit, or in this case, the cause of your vasoconstriction.

First, look for the stimulus. What has just occurred in your environment that conceivably could have been the S in the SAD sequence? Try to piece together what possible thought processes or self-statements could have been going on that led to the conclusion that your life or limb has been threatened and/or that a law of nature has been violated. You can check out several hypotheses in order to determine what this analysis may have consisted of. You can actually say to yourself, "Did I use the word *should* in relation to the stimulus?" You could also query yourself to find out if you made the event seem catastrophic or used the word *need*. You know you will have adequately solved the crime when you can put together an analysis that fits all the facts. The final proof, of course, comes when you have reanalyzed the stimulus and no longer react to it as though it were a danger signal. The more persistent a detective you become, the more likely it is that those vasoconstrictions will cease to cause you trouble.

My thinking on the causes and treatment of danger signals has been heavily influenced by a psychologist, Dr. Albert Ellis. Dr. Ellis has developed a self-help system of therapy for dealing with emotional upsets. He believes that almost everybody suffers unnecessarily from emotional reactions to events that go on in the world around them. Dr. Ellis extensively treats the thought processes that lead one to become upset. For those of you who would like additional material on how to deal with SADs, I would highly recommend the book, *Guide to Rational Living*, by Dr. Ellis.

Combining the use of vasodilation and SAD reanalysis skills

I have been stressing the usefulness of becoming aware of vasoconstrictions so that you can identify SADs and reanalyze them. In a previous chapter, I also emphasized the benefits of becoming aware of vasoconstrictions and how you can use this awareness as a signal that it is time for you to practice a vasodilation skill. Therefore, at this point, it is perhaps a little unclear as to what you should do first, once you have noticed that a vasoconstriction has occurred. Should you first do the preventive maintenance, practicing a vasodilation skill, or should you first use the vasoconstriction as a signal that it is time to identify a SAD?

I actually would like to see you do both. That is, when a vasoconstriction has occurred and you notice it, the first thing to do is say "vasodilate" to yourself and very briefly attempt to reverse the vasoconstrictive process. By briefly, I mean in not more than one or two minutes. You may or may not be successful at this particular point in reversing the vasoconstriction. Whether you are or not, however, after you have made this brief attempt, it is time to begin an identification of the SAD that might have just occurred.

I suggest that you follow this particular order once a vasoconstriction has occurred because the primary prevention technique for
migraine headaches is to stop a vasoconstriction. Once you have
vasoconstricted, it is important to try and reverse this condition. I
believe that at that particular time, the best chance you have of
reversing vasoconstriction is to practice your vasodilation skills.
However, the SAD might be so strong you might not be able to
overcome it by voluntary vasodilation. If that is the case, the vasoconstriction could perhaps be best eliminated by an SAD analysis. In
the long run, the SAD analysis will perhaps also prevent future such
occurrences when a similar S is presented again.

The primary prevention technique for migraine headaches is to stop a vasoconstriction.

There is one additional advantage in attempting to briefly vasodilate before you do your SAD analysis. Doing a SAD analysis really
requires a great deal of thought which in turn requires a rich blood
supply to the higher thinking centers in your brain. If you are vasoconstricted, your thinking will not be as efficient. By attempting a
brief vasodilation after a SAD has occurred and before you actually
begin the SAD reanalysis, the chances are you will increase the blood
supply to the higher centers of your brain and make the SAD reanalysis an easier task.

In any event, I wish to repeat my observation made in the previous section. You are not a perfect human being and you will not be
able to reverse all vasoconstrictions and do SAD reanalyses in an
ideal manner. There will be times when you will totally forget even
to attempt a vasodilation or SAD reanalysis, much less do it according to the book. The reality is that you will do what you can and are
ready to do at the particular time. Allow yourself the privilege of not
being perfect, of not doing the best you can and in fact doing, at
times, a rather poor and mediocre job. The techniques and procedures that I have been suggesting in this book are worthwhile ones
and will help you to overcome your headache pain. Since I believe
this, I also am convinced that whatever you can do, it is an improvement and better than not doing anything at all.

**For those patients who feel their headaches are not connected to
danger signals in the world around them**

The following session recently took place in my office with a patient
who had begun my migraine treatment program three weeks before.
Up to the previous weekend, she had been absolutely delighted with
her progress since she had not had a headache for two weeks which
was, for this particular woman, the longest headache-free period
that she had had in years. That Sunday night, however, she began to
feel that mild tenseness around the back of her neck which is the
signal that she is about to begin a severe migraine headache. Within
two hours, her headache followed its usual course and became an

extremely excruciating pain in her left side that totally disabled her.

She said that she had not done her Medlaxing on that Sunday. Although contrary to my instructions, she felt she could forego Medlaxing since it had been an extremely delightful and low pressure day. Further, she insisted that there were no tigers leaping out at her that could have produced vasoconstriction and then led to her headache.

She described her day as follows: After toast and coffee, she and her husband went to the church they had been going to for many years. My patient told me that she finds church a relaxing experience, and after this particular service, found it even more enjoyable since they remained for a social gathering and had a chance to drink some coffee and visit people whom they haven't had a chance to talk to in some time. There were no negative conversations that she could recall.

After church, they went home and had a brunch and then visited her husband's uncle who lived in a home for the aged across town. That visit also went well, and old Uncle Fred was happy to see both of them. Following their visit to Uncle Fred, they went shopping for groceries and for a new suit for her husband. In the evening they visited with their children and grandchildren, who came over to their house for dessert. All in all, she described it as one of the better days of the week and could certainly see no reason for vasoconstricting. As I inquired further, however, it turned out that several "tigers" were encountered on this seemingly innocuous day.

To begin with, it is important to realize that my patient, whom I consider to be an absolutely delightful woman, had one glaring *should* that led to many danger signals throughout her daily life. She felt that she *should* visit, call, and talk to old friends on a regular, perhaps weekly basis. She felt it was neglectful and inconsiderate of others, particularly her friends, if she did not do so. She was convinced that her friends would think that she didn't care for them anymore if she didn't maintain this regular contact.

This *should* was further extended to family members, particularly those who did not have a lot of contact with other people, such as her husband's uncle in the nursing home. There are, of course, limits, to how much any one individual can do within a twenty-four-hour day, and my patient was deluged with activities which ranged from volunteer work to a major remodeling job in her home. In addition, she and her husband had been working in their summer home whenever they had available time to get it ready for the up-coming season. Consequently, she had not been doing the amount of visiting and calling and maintaining contact with her friends that she felt she *should* be doing.

At some level, my patient probably thought that her friends felt slighted and that she didn't like them anymore. So, although she certainly enjoyed meeting some of these friends at the church coffee hour, they also were a stimulus for a SAD sequence since she was reminded of how negligent she had been. She was reminded that she wasn't doing what she *should* have been doing in terms of her self-imposed law of nature regarding obligations to friends.

This seemingly innocuous church coffee hour became an occasion for my patient's arteries to constrict and thus set her up for a possible migraine headache.

However, she probably shouldn't have developed a migraine headache from this small amount of vasoconstriction, but compounded with a visit to her husband's uncle later on, some additional vasoconstriction was added to that already present. Again, although the visit seemed to go well, she felt that she had been negligent in not keeping up her visitations to this elderly gentleman. Even though she had visited him in the past perhaps even more than closer relatives had been doing, she felt that her other activities should not have interfered with these visits.

So, here we have two seemingly innocuous visits that, because of her analysis, led to vasoconstrictions. Once again, these two may not have led to a migraine headache. However, she also had the evening with her children and grandchildren (which she typically enjoys) but she probably needed to be alone that night because of the strains of the day. Needless to say, added together all of the vasoconstrictions were sufficient to bring on her headache.

Two things could have happened during the day, either one of which might have prevented the onset of my patient's headache. First, she could have regularly used the Medlax, which would have overcome or reduced the amount of vasoconstriction in her arteries. Second, if she knew she was vasoconstricting, she could have done a reanalysis of the SAD sequence and prevented her danger signals.

In the future, hopefully my patient will be more sensitive to her own bodily reactions and to those situations that produce vasoconstrictions, so that she can perhaps avoid most of her headaches. This is a good illustration of why it is important to keep up with regular Medlaxing even though you may feel there is no reason for your arteries to have constricted. Medlaxing takes only a few minutes during the day, whereas the amount of time lost due to head pain, not to mention the extreme discomfort and unpleasantness of it all, may last many hours, even days.

Time and time again, I have run into conflict with my patients over the idea that vasoconstrictions are brought about by seemingly innocuous or unimportant daily events. I would like to emphasize that I am not suggesting that you are more psychologically disturbed than anyone else in the population. You are, however, much more apt to react to minor disturbances with a vasoconstriction than seems to be the case with most other people.

It is very possible to look at your disorder, overreactive arteries, as a mixed blessing. On the one hand, they are precisely the cause of

I am not suggesting that you are more psychologically disturbed than anyone else in the population.

In a sense, you have a greater opportunity to improve the quality of your life than might be possible if you were not afflicted with migraine headaches.

your migraine headaches. On the other hand, your reactive arteries can be used to your benefit to allow you to be more sensitive to your own body and its reactions to potentially upsetting situations. Whereas those who do not suffer from migraines may not show any symptoms in reaction to these situations, they are getting upset whether they are aware of it or not. Changes are going on somewhere in their bodies, but fortunately for them, at least in this stage of their life, they do not exhibit any symptoms. You, however, have the opportunity to make things better by looking more carefully at those situations that produce vasoconstrictions and perhaps changing the way that you view them or altering the situations themselves. In a sense, you have a greater opportunity to improve the quality of your life than might be possible if you were not afflicted with migraine headaches.

SADs that don't go away

If you are unsuccessful in reducing or eliminating the occurrence of SADs through the approach given in this chapter, this could mean that you need professional help in accomplishing your goal. There are times when our own personal biases and perceptions prevent us from objectively analyzing our own thoughts and behavior. A professional psychotherapist can be more objective about your problems and can be in a good position to help you see things from a different viewpoint.

Migraine pain as a danger signal

From reading this book, you know that I feel your migraine headaches are caused by vasoconstrictions in the arteries supplying blood to your brain. You also know that I have suggested that this reaction can be changed through the use of biofeedback and relaxation skills. In this chapter I have pointed out that how you analyze the world around you is also important in understanding and controlling your headaches.

A patient to whom I once explained these very same theories suddenly broke into tears and in a sobbing voice said, "I knew these headaches were my fault. I shouldn't be having them and causing my family so much trouble." Not all migraine sufferers feel responsible for their headaches, but if you are one of them, don't blame yourself. A migraine headache is a painful and discouraging experience. It is truly unfortunate that many migraine suffers tend to make their pain even worse by getting emotionally upset at the fact that they have migraines when they believe that they shouldn't.

Notice the use of the word *shouldn't*. If you believe you *should not* be having migraine headaches, then of course every time you have one you are giving your body the signal that a law of nature has been violated. Your analysis will lead you to make a very difficult and painful situation even worse. Hopefully, by following the techniques that I have outlined in this book, you can start using the laws of nature (controlling arteries) to do something to avoid these painful experiences.

Basically, I am pleading with you to allow yourself to be imperfect and to not upset yourself more than you have to when you have a migraine headache. Nobody is perfect, and the methods that I discuss in this book are not perfect either. Do the best you can, but if you can't, then allow yourself to do a mediocre or incomplete job. I believe the techniques in this book are worthwhile doing on even a mediocre and infrequent basis. I prefer, of course, that you diligently follow the schedule and the techniques as outlined. But I also understand that migraine sufferers, like everyone else in the world, are humans who are far from perfect.

Do the best you can, but if you can't, allow yourself to do a mediocre or incomplete job.

Now that you have read this far—

Now that you have read this far, I will briefly review the suggestions that I have made to help you eliminate or reduce your migraine pain:

1. Using the biotic band, try to raise your finger temperature as much as possible within a three- to four-minute period at least three to four times each day. Remember to say "vasodilate" to yourself before each attempt at biofeedback, as well as before each Medlax practice.
2. In order to improve your awareness of finger temperature (and vasoconstrictions), guess what your finger temperature is before you read the biotic band.
3. Practice the Medlax at least every other hour during your waking day.
4. When you notice that a vasoconstriction has occurred or that you have become emotionally upset, first say "vasodilate" to yourself and briefly attempt to use whatever vasodilation skills you have to stop and reverse the vasoconstriction. Second, look for and reanalyze the SAD.

6

ONE FINAL STEP IN AVOIDING VASOCONSTRICTIONS

Early in this book, I suggested that one of the ways you can avoid vasoconstrictions is to not go out into the world seeking "tigers." As illogical as this seems, the chances are that you *do* seek tigers. And when you discover them, they produce a danger signal which in turn produces a vasoconstriction. There are enough tigers lying out there in the bushes ready to spring up at us without our actually having to go out and beat the bushes to produce even more of them. In fact, we can even avoid walking in the woods in the first place, which certainly makes sense if we are trying to avoid wild animals. The tigers and animals I am talking about, of course, are those day-to-day danger signals that come from dealing with bosses, children, spouses, workloads, finances, deadlines, etc.

Assert yourself—saying no to a tiger

Suppose a friend came up to you and said, "I would like you to take a walk in that forest over yonder and see if any tigers happen to jump out at you. I know you are busy, but I'd sure appreciate it." There is a very important behavior that can be used in this situation to guarantee the avoidance of a vasoconstriction. All you have to do is say, "No." Chances are that you would say no if a friend really did request you to go out and provoke a tiger. Saying no, however, is extremely difficult for many people.

Now suppose your friend instead said to you, "I know you're very busy, but I would greatly appreciate if you could go door-to-door to the homes in your neighborhood to work for the Children's Hospital Guild. It is such a worthy charity, you know, since it helps all of those poor unfortunate children who would be without hope except for your efforts." Assuming that you are busy and truly do not want to do this type of door-to-door solicitation, instead of saying, "No," you might say "... I'm really not very good at going door-to-door and . . . uh . . . people don't give very much when I do it and I think that . . . uh . . . I really must stay home and be with my two children, they're only two and three you see and. . . ."

Your friend then might say, "Oh, that's all right; I know that you will do the best you can and whatever you do is okay. It's perfectly okay to take your children with you, the fresh air will do them good and it's really nice to get out of the house. So I'll drop off the pledge cards to you. I really appreciate your kindness."

At this point it's probably even more difficult for you to say no than it would have been in the first place, so you reluctantly consent. I can assure you that sometime during the next day, as you are trying to do your household chores and you notice that it is getting too late to go out collecting, you will probably have a vasoconstriction and will remain in that vasoconstricted state till you have adequately resolved your dilemma in one way or another. If only you would have said no in the first place, you probably would have avoided one and possibly more migraine headaches.

In recent years there has been a great deal of attention given to this problem of saying no. Several books and many articles have been written on saying no. The problem is overcome by learning how to become assertive. If you are assertive you will express your feelings and desires and avoid being in the woods unnecessarily.

In order to learn how to become assertive, you need to understand why you are so reluctant to say the word *no* in the first place. There are really very good reasons for this problem. In the short-term, it is probably even to your benefit to not be assertive. If you are assertive and say no to a request made of you, there may be a few minutes, or perhaps even hours of being upset and uncomfortable.

The short-term benefit of not being assertive, then, is that you avoid those uncomfortable feelings. In the long-term, however, you clearly pay the price for not being assertive. The long-term discomfort from vasoconstriction far outweighs the short-term discomfort which you avoid by saying yes to something when you could say no.

> The long-term discomfort from vasoconstriction far outweighs the short-term discomfort which you avoid by saying yes when you could say no.

In the previous chapter, I discussed the SAD sequence. When you say yes, you are often avoiding an immediate S in a SAD sequence. Let me give you an example by referring back to your friend who asked you to collect for a charitable cause. Let's say you have not yet done a SAD reanalysis. Chances are that if you had said no, this would have been an S in an SAD sequence. Very soon after saying no you probably would have experienced a danger signal due to your analysis (A) of the situation. Your analysis probably would have gone something like this: "I said no to my friend; she will probably no longer like me. She will be angry with me and think that I am selfish. *I need to be liked and thought well of by her at all times.* Since I am not getting what I *need*, my life is being threatened."

As unreasonable as this line of thinking seems to be, we all engage in one form or another of it from time to time. We know we engage in this kind of thinking because our arteries vasoconstrict. Since they vasoconstrict, we know that a danger signal has occurred. Since a danger signal has occurred, we have concluded that there has been a threat to our life or that a law of nature has been violated. So by saying yes instead of no we have avoided a SAD—temporarily.

The kicker, of course, is that by avoiding one SAD we are then presented with another. The replacement puts us in a situation with a great many time demands requiring behavior (collecting from neighbors) that is difficult for us to perform. Once in this situation, we then proceed to analyze it in a way that invariably will produce a danger signal. I am not as concerned with this second SAD as I am with the first. If you do a reanalysis of your first SAD, you might be in a position to say no and not experience a danger signal, hence avoiding any SAD whatsoever.

Let me give you some of the self-statements and thinking that lead to an analysis of saying no which produces a danger signal for us. By looking closely at this type of thinking, we can see how unreasonable it is and replace it with a different and more appropriate analysis, thus avoiding feeling uncomfortable and experiencing the danger signal.

One idea is that you *should* not say no to a request that is made of you. Notice the use of the word *should* as though a law of nature were being stated. This kind of thinking is generally acquired as we are growing up under the influence of our parents. To a small child, parents are all-powerful, know everything, and have only noble intentions. Further, to a small child, being in the good graces of a parent truly is a matter of life or death. When we are very small we do not have the means to provide for and take care of ourselves. A parent who is angry has the power to abandon us.

Don't get me wrong; I'm not down on parents. I'm just saying that they are human beings like everyone else and are subject to the neuroses and erroneous A analyses that every human being experiences. As loving, concerned, and fair as a parent may be, saying no to their requests can often be met with their disfavor. To the child, this disfavor can be blown out of proportion and interpreted as a matter of survival. This "training" means that you enter adulthood with a fairly automatic SAD reaction. When you even contemplate saying no to a request, you begin to experience the vasoconstriction and discomfort that come from being presented with a danger signal.

You can overcome these automatic reactions by going through the steps outlined in the previous chapter. When you notice that you would like to say no to a request and you begin to experience discomfort and a vasoconstriction, say to yourself that a danger signal or SAD sequence has just taken place. Identify the stimulus, which in this case will be the request made by somebody and your desire to say no. Then proceed to discover what your analysis is that is leading to a danger signal. Look for the use of the words *should* and *need* in order to find out why you have concluded your analysis with the notion that a law of nature has been violated or that there is a threat to your life or limb.

Once you have discovered what your analysis is, begin your reanalysis by changing key words and saying to yourself that your life is not being endangered or that a law of nature has not been violated. I know that this reanalysis might be very difficult to perform, particularly if a vasoconstriction has already occurred and you are not thinking as clearly as you would like to. It is possible, however, that after you have said yes and had time to think about it, after your reanalysis, you can get back to that individual and change your yes to a no.

Do not expect yourself to suddenly change from a yes-saying person to a no-saying person by simply reading this chapter. It will take some concerted effort on your part. It would be nice if you could begin to work on this problem today. In time, saying no to those things that you do not wish to become involved with or do not want will be as second nature to you as eating and breathing.

I also want you to keep in mind that even if you have said yes when you would have preferred to say no, you can still use the SAD analysis to help you not overreact and vasoconstrict when you end up doing a task that you really wish you didn't have to do. This actually is the second line of defense for avoiding unnecessary vasoconstrictions. However, the emphasis in this chapter is on the first line of defense, allowing you to get to the point where you can say no and not experience an emotional upset or vasoconstriction as a result of asserting your rights.

Aggression and assertion

There is an important distinction between being assertive and being aggressive. Assertion is simply standing up for your rights and doing what you happen to think is correct for yourself at that particular time. With a thorough analysis of SADs, you can expect to learn to be assertive without experiencing any discomfort or vasoconstrictions.

Aggression is quite different. Rather than just asserting your rights, or standing up for what you believe to be correct and appropriate, aggression involves the use of hostility with an intent to hurt the other individual. Aggression is usually the result, incidentally, of an inappropriate analysis of a situation that leads us to perceive a danger signal to which we react with a fighting response. This fighting, or aggression, response is typically just as avoidable by reanalysis as any other danger signal.

There is one other aspect of assertion that really doesn't center around the use of the word no but is also very important. This involves telling an individual how you felt about a particular action or activity that resulted in discomfort for you. For example, let us assume that you are a nonsmoker who does not wish to be exposed to the smoke generated by someone who is sitting next to you at a lunch counter. Everyone has the right to express his or her feelings and to tell someone else that their behavior is bothersome. If you are to be assertive in this situation, you tell the individual next to you that the smoke bothers you and ask that the cigarette be put out or that the individual move to a different section of the counter where there are other smokers.

If you are not assertive and do not feel you have the right to express your feelings, even contemplating such a minor situation results in a SAD. Faulty analysis will tell you that you *should* not offend another person, nor should you take the chance of having the other person not think well of you because you *need* to be thought well of by everybody all the time. By doing a reanalysis, you can discover that this is not a life or death situation, nor is it a situation in which there will be a violation of a law of nature. There will then be no vasoconstriction or emotional upset and your feelings can be directly expressed.

If your faulty analysis includes ideas like "That smoker *should* not be smoking here and *should* be more considerate of other people," then you will manufacture and present to yourself a danger signal which will result in vasoconstriction and perhaps a feeling of anger. You might lose your temper instead of expressing your feelings in a direct and calm manner. You might even become aggressive and indignant in your response. In any event, by being assertive and expressing your feelings, there is a chance, sometimes very good, that the other individual will willingly oblige you and thus remove a stimulus that could lead to a danger signal.

Assertions involving expressions of feelings and preferences are extremely important in relationships that occur with spouses, children, colleagues, employees, etc. By letting such individuals know what you would like and what you would prefer in an assertive but nonaggressive way, you can eliminate a large number of "tigers" that you may have been running into on a daily basis, perhaps for years. There are enough tigers in this world that are difficult to send away, so I strongly urge you to use assertion to get rid of those that can be so easily eliminated.

Time management and perfectionism

In order to help you say no to another type of tiger lurking in the bushes, I want to address two seemingly unconnected topics. These two, time management and perfectionism, often plague migraine sufferers. So many of my migraine patients complain about not hav-ing enough time to do all of the things that they would like. They have so many different things to do that it seems the day goes by, and perhaps even the night, and they're left with the uneasy feeling that they have just begun to scratch the surface. My patients with these time problems then begin to worry and fret over what must be done the next day in order to not only do the next day's jobs but also make up for what they didn't do today. The more these tasks seem to accumulate, the more rushed and hurried my patients become and, you guessed it, the more vasoconstricted their arteries become also.

Time management problems and perfectionism often plague migraine sufferers.

Time management is a method by which individuals can use the hours that they have available to accomplish what it is they would like to do. It is based on the idea that everybody seems to have the same amount of time, yet some people tend to accomplish those things that they want done in a given period while others al-ways seem to be falling behind.

One well-known time management expert gives the following two "rules of time management" to those of us who are not accom-plishing what we would like to in a given period of time.

The First Rule of Time Management

It is important to decide which are the most important activities. That is, of all the things you would like to do, which have the high-est priority for you? This perhaps sounds easier to do than it actually is. It perhaps seems to many of us that everything is important and everything has high priority. It certainly is important to return a phone call that may have come in to you, and it certainly is impor-tant to drive the car pool and pick up the children when it is your turn, and it certainly is important to get your bid in on time on that large project, and it certainly is important to pay the electric bill and the house payment on time.

Here is how you can go about placing a priority on each of the various kinds of tasks that confront you. One little trick will actually help you considerably to master this particular problem. Take about ten minutes, sit down at a table with some paper and a pencil and try to make sure that your ten-minute period of time will be undis-turbed so you can think without distractions.

First write down what it is that you would like to have accom-plished in your life one year from now. Do the same thing for six months and five years from now. List all the various goals that you might have. They might be interpersonal goals such as an improved relationship with your wife or the acquisition of some new friends or learning how to overcome shyness when you're with a group of strangers. They might be financial goals such as preparing yourself to move up in your company to a more prestigious and higher paying position or saving $1,000 or paying off a large balance that has been running some time on your bank card statement. On the other hand some of your goals might be more quality-of-life and recreation oriented. For example, you might wish to change your living conditions.

Once you have decided what your overall goals are, you can then look at them and decide which are the most important for you to accomplish. I suggest that you use the star system to signify the importance of your various goals. Five stars might be the most important goals you wish to accomplish, whereas one-star goals, although desired by you, are considerably less important than a three-star or two-star goal.

Now that you have set priorities on your longer-term goals, you can think about your next day's activities to see which of your next day's activities will help you to accomplish your six-month, one-year and five-year goals. By looking at longer-term goals, you can gain perspective on day-to-day activities. You are now in a position to rank the importance of day-to-day activities in relation to your long-term goals. Of course the question now arises, once you have ranked importance, what do you do? Does this mean you won't do anything that doesn't lead to long-term goals and only focus on those activities that in fact will help you toward this end? No, unfortunately many tasks on a day-to-day basis are desirable even though they are not directly related to long-term accomplishments. There is, however, another important technique that you can use in conjunction with the knowledge of importance that will help you to make the maximum use of your time.

The Second Rule of Time Management

The second rule of time management is don't do a high quality or perfect job on those things that are least important in accomplishing long-term goals. It makes perfectly good sense, when you think about it, not to waste your time doing a high quality job on some task that really doesn't require it. I know that for many of my patients, this is much easier said than done. The reason that my patients have difficulty in following this advice is that they are perfectionists. Your own desires and beliefs that you must be perfect, or at least everything that you do should be the best job possible or as close to perfection as one can achieve stands in the way of your accomplishing long-term goals and managing time in such a way as to avoid vasoconstrictions.

Perfectionism—the Mixed Blessing

"If you can't do a job well, then don't do it at all."

These words ring like chimes of truth that seem so obvious to many of my patients that they have never, even once, questioned their ultimate wisdom.

I challenge the validity of this saying even though I am aware that nearly everyone appreciates a job well done. For example, I am particularly proud of a small wooden sailing pram that I recently acquired. It is truly finished to perfection. The copper nails are all countersunk and the small openings left by these nails have been filled in with wooden plugs. The entire surface has been sanded and filled so that the finished product has an almost mirror-like quality. When I show this boat to my friends, I point to it and speak glowingly of the two brothers who build these boats in a manner that one associates with an era long past. It is difficult to find such workmanship and perfection in today's products. Correspondingly, these two boat builders have all the work they can possibly handle, and it is necessary to place your order almost a year in advance. Perfectionism has certainly paid off for these two.

Nine months after ordering my boat, I was finally notified that it was ready. At the time that I picked it up at their small island boatyard, they invited me into their business office to complete the necessary financial arrangements before the boat was truly mine. The office was located adjacent to the boat-building shop, so that we had to walk through the work area to get to the office. The shop itself didn't look like an ordinary carpenter's shop at all. Everything was in its place, and there was practically no sawdust on the floor. Vacuum spouts with hoses were located at strategic points and apparently continuously used in order to maintain the spotless appearance of the work area. As we passed through the entrance leading from the shop into the office I looked about in disbelief. Here was a jumble of papers, records, books, and broken wooden chairs on which I had to balance myself to avoid falling.

A spot was cleared on the desk so that I could have a surface flat enough on which to write out my check and for the brothers to make out their receipt. The receipt book, incidentally, was found with much difficulty under a boating magazine and a catalogue for plumbing fixtures (I didn't know what that was doing there). After our business was completed, I simply had to ask them why there was such great contrast between their office and record system and their boat shop with its neat, tidy appearance and well-organized layout.

Both the brothers chuckled at my observation and said simply that for them, building boats was important, and further they wanted to build the best boat that was possible. Recordkeeping, business matters were relatively unimportant and were a nuisance that could easily result in a lot of wasted time. They spoke disdainfully of a fellow boat builder who used to live down the road. He had spread his energy too thin because he attempted not only to build perfect boats but also to run a first-class business office. Eventually, he had to hire a bookkeeper which in turn necessitated employing other master carpenters to help build volume to meet his higher overhead expenses. He builds lots of boats, they say, but he is unhappy with the product and is constantly working overtime trying to perfect and correct the work of others, as well as putting in additional time in the office to make sure records are in order. They figured that in about a year he would either have a mental breakdown, or be out of business.

Let us compare the perfectionism of the brothers to the other boat contractor. The difference between the doomed boat builder down the road and the two brothers was that efforts at perfectionism were controlled and focused in one case and in the other were diffuse and applied to every aspect of the business. The lesson to be learned is straightforward. Perfectionism has its payoffs, but used to extreme it can lead to stress and failure.

I know this conclusion seems obvious and sensible. Most everybody would agree that it is foolish to try to be perfect in everything that one does because such a goal is impossible to attain and by necessity, limits the number and type of activities in which one can engage. Even though it makes sense, I'm fully aware that if you are unfortunate enough to try being perfectionist at a great many things, it is extremely difficult to change this way of approaching life. The difficulty comes not because you don't know *how* to be imperfect or *how* to do a job in a mediocre manner; the difficulty comes from the emotional upset that you feel when a job is less than perfect.

For some people it's downright unsettling to leave their desk without putting everything away neatly or to do an architectural drawing that may have some smudges or irregular lines or to prepare a report for internal circulation only that has a mistake of no great consequence here and there. The dishes that have not been put away, the towels that have not been hung neatly or the newspaper that has been left lying on the floor—all of these little events, which would have no consequence on the quality of your life or achievement of your goals, are reacted to as though a danger signal had been presented. The perfectionist has the experience of tension or anxiety, a gnawing feeling that something bad is about to occur, unless everything is done just right. The rules, "it *must* be done right," "it *must* be done properly," "it *must* be done perfectly," are burned into your thinking. You have accepted these rules as laws of nature, and if they are violated, you feel that horrible things are going to happen.

Perfectionism can be extremely destructive and lead to many unnecessary SADs during daily activities. SADs occur after you have completed a job, let's say cleaned the house, and you look at it and see that things are not quite in order. A speck of thread is on the floor, a spot of dust is on the bookcase, there are some cups and saucers yet to be put away. When you are tempted to leave this stimulus situation, a danger signal is quickly presented—because you

Perfectionism has its payoffs, but used to extreme it can lead to stress and failure.

have analyzed this situation (a job not complete or done perfectly) as though it were a threat to life or limb or as though a law of nature has been violated.

As I have pointed out, our analysis leads us to these conclusions because we have somewhere learned that a job should be perfect. You probably learned this perfectionism very early in life from your parents who became upset or unhappy with you as a child when you didn't do things just right. To the child, a parent being upset seems like a direct threat to life or limb. In reality, people rarely do the best job that they can do, much less a perfect job.

Before you can effectively begin to manage time by doing some jobs much less than perfectly and other jobs at a barely adequate level, it is important to reanalyze any SADs that may occur when you are confronted with your mediocre work. I am clearly suggesting to you that you purposely *not* do a good job (and certainly *not* a perfect one) on most of the tasks that you have to perform. Expend your energy and efforts and perfectionism only on high-priority activities. These are the activities that you have previously determined will help you accomplish the things that are most important in your life.

I am clearly suggesting to you that you *not* do a good job (and certainly *not* a perfect one) on most of the tasks that you have to perform.

Perfectionism is not easy to overcome if it has been a life-long habit. I suggest that you work at it. Purposely leave a job half done or inadequately done. You'll find that no law of nature has been violated, nor will your life or limb be threatened. Once you see that nothing terrible or bad will happen when you do mediocre work, you can use the time management principles of only putting in high quality work on those items which will help you to accomplish your longer-term goals. Furthermore not only are some jobs best done on a mediocre or barely adequate level, some can even be put off until the next day or even the next week. Some may not ever have to be done at all.

Not only are some jobs best done on a mediocre or barely adequate level, some can even be put off until the next day or even the next week. Some may not ever have to be done at all.

Again, to accomplish this noble goal of doing mediocre work will require you to do a careful analysis of the SADs that occur when the job is done much less than adequately. By carefully analyzing, you can avoid the vasoconstrictions and consequent migraine headaches, while at the same time accomplish more. Becoming less than a perfectionist will help you accomplish more in one other very significant way: By not being so insistent on perfection and so exposing yourself to unnecessary SADs, you can avoid some of the pain and lost time that accrues from those headaches that you have overcome.

Worrying

"If only I could stop this incessant worrying over every detail and everything that has gone wrong and what I think is going to go wrong, my life would be so different."

Worrying is a problem for the migraine sufferer because as you go over all of the details and thoughts that are contained in a so-called problem you will inevitably produce some thoughts or ideas that are SADs.

There are actually two different approaches that I use with my patients I consider to be excessive worriers. The first involves determining whether or not the worrying is functional. That is, is the worrying beneficial or not beneficial? Excessive worrying, incidentally, is rarely beneficial. I think that worrying occurs very often because, at times, it is very useful to plan, contemplate, or rehearse various thoughts in one's mind so that you will not repeat an error that has been made in the past or will know how to deal with an upcoming situation when it does occur.

For example, I am writing this chapter on the way to catching a ferry for one of the islands which so beautifully dot the waters in the Pacific Northwest. I had to do a considerable amount of thinking and worrying about the time that I should get up, making sure that my alarm clock was set properly and worked, rehearsing the route that I would follow and taking care of some errands and other arrangements that were necessary before I could leave for the day. I am, incidentally, on the way to give a lecture on the use of biofeedback in clinical practice to a community mental health clinic which is located on one of the islands. I point this out because from time to time patients have told me that if they could only get away from the city life and live in a more relaxed manner in one of these idyllic settings they would not have any problems. Their stresses would disappear and so would their symptoms and dissatisfactions.

Well, this island I am visiting is inhabited by just such souls. A large portion of the population are runaways from the urban life. I don't know what the statistics are precisely, expect that the community mental health center is as busy here in attempting to deal with stress-related problems as are similar facilities located in the midst of heavily populated, noisy, and polluted cities. It seems that SADs occur wherever the person happens to be since the manner in which a person analyzes stimuli will not change with his location.

In any event, a certain amount of planning, forethought and perhaps even rehashing of things that have gone wrong can be useful. The fact that such planning *can* be useful is the reason why we learned how to do this worrying in the first place. The problem, of course, is that the "worrier" goes far beyond what is functional. Worries will plague the person every day for hours at a time and interfere with participating in what is going on at the moment in the world that surrounds the individual. So, I suggest that you give yourself permission to do a certain amount of this functional worrying, but be well aware that most of this kind of activity is not useful and, in fact, can lead to danger signals which will lead to vasoconstrictions and eventually migraines.

The second approach I use with individuals who worry runs counter to intuition. I do not think you should try to get rid of these thoughts that plague you by attempting to put them out of your mind. Instead you should extend your worrying so that you can spell out the eventual results or consequences of what it is that you are worrying about.

For example, one of my patients was worried about the possibility that he would look like a fool when he had to present to a group of coworkers and supervisors a summary of his progress on a particular project. He did not consider himself to be a good public speaker, and this presentation was to be done orally. He also felt he had not done as well as he *should* have done on this project and was certain that the listeners to his presentation would be able to see this. Although this presentation was two weeks off, he constantly ruminated and imagined in his mind how he was going to give the talk and what he would say. He kept going over the same scenarios again and again and again and, in fact, knew pretty well exactly what it was that he was going to say even before he began this incessant worrying. So his worrying was no longer functional and, in fact, was producing vasoconstrictions which conceivably could even result in a migraine headache that would interfere with the presentation itself.

Here is the advice that I gave to this particular patient. First assess the probabilities that various types of bad or embarrassing outcomes could occur. Is there a fifty-fifty chance that you will be frozen with anxiety and not be able to speak? Or is it a ninety-ten chance? Or is there such small probability that this will happen that it is even hard to anticipate? What are the chances that people will laugh at some mistake?

It is important to make these probability assessments since we very often worry about extremely improbable events. It is extremely improbable, for example, that we will be hit and killed by a car as we walk across the street at any particular time. Given that this is such a low probability, often recognizing the unlikelihood of it occurring is sufficient to stop worrying. But let us assume you have assessed the probabilities of unpleasant events actually occurring, and even if they are low, you still continue to worry.

It is at this point that I asked my patient to extend his worrying one step beyond what most worriers actually do. What if the unpleasant event actually occurs, i.e., what if you forget certain important facts and figures during the talk or mix them up so that it doesn't make much sense? What then would happen? It is, of course, at this point that an S of an SAD series is presented and, depending on what your analysis of the situation is, will determine whether or not a danger signal gets presented. If you conclude it will be a catastrophe, i.e., you will be immediately fired and no longer be able to provide food and shelter for yourself and your family, then a danger signal will be presented to your body and a vasoconstriction will occur. If your analysis is more reasonable, however, you will not feel that it will be catastrophe and you should always be perfect. Further, you will recognize and tell yourself that even though some people may not think highly of you at that particular moment, it doesn't mean they always will think poorly of you. Most important, of course, is that your reanalysis will not permit the conclusion that a life threatening event or law of nature has been violated. You will not vasoconstrict, and your actual performance during your oral presentation will be at its best since the maximum amount of blood possible will be flowing into the cortex of your brain so that you can think clearly, have the best memory that you can, and be able to handle emergency or unexpected situations in an optimal way.

My advice to worriers is, after you have decided whether or not your worrying is functional or dysfunctional, take your dysfunctional worries and try to actually imagine the consequences of what it is that you are worried about. At that point, reanalyze so that your SAD disappears.

Worrying over Being Late

In my practice, I see patients who suffer from a wide variety of disorders. For some their primary complaint is pain in their lower back. For others, it might be a nervous stomach or colitis. For others it might be excessive fear. Everybody is different, and I do not like to identify a particular symptom with a personality type. Even though I have reservations about saying that a person with hypertension, for example, feels frustrated and is overly ambitious, there are times when certain behaviors seem to go with certain kinds of physical and medical problems. For example, I expect tardiness from my patients who have symptoms like hypertension, tension headaches, ulcers, etc., but I am always taken by surprise when a migraine patient is late for an appointment. Although I admit I certainly like my patients to show up on time for appointments, I am somewhat dismayed when I hear about a patient's extreme amount of worrying and planning in order to assure *always, absolutely always*, being on time for an appointment. When you worry and fret and plan so that you will always be on time, you no doubt are going to produce unnecessary vasoconstrictions and render yourself vulnerable to a migraine headache.

A patient recently showed up five minutes late and had what I can best describe as a look of terror on her face. She explained to me that she knew I was a very busy man and that she felt just terrible showing up late for this appointment. She further enumerated the various precautions that she had taken to make sure that such a terrible thing could not happen. Unfortunately an emergency had occurred at her office which delayed her over thirty minutes. She found the emergency very stressful to deal with, but in addition was extremely upset over the fact that she might be late for her appointment. She told me that "she is always on time," and hates it when she is late or if anybody else is late for an appointment with her.

Up to this point, this particular patient had been making considerable progress in overcoming her migraine headaches as indicated by the temperature measurements that we had obtained on her fingers in the office. Over the past several weeks she had shown an overall increase of 15 degrees in her fingertip temperature. On this day, the day that she was late, however, her fingertip temperature was at the initial, low reading she had when she first began treatment. After obtaining some temperature and muscle tension measurements on this patient, I decided not to continue with the biofeedback but instead to discuss the SAD sequence that had led to her vasoconstriction.

The stimulus, S, was coming late for an appointment. Her analysis, A, was based on an erroneous law of nature that she had adopted in her own mind. The erroneous law of nature was that she "*should* always be on time for an appointment." Since this law of nature had been violated, a danger signal, D, was presented and she showed a vasoconstriction.

Let us do a reanalysis of this stimulus. First, there is no law of nature that says one should always be on time for an appointment. In fact any law of nature which takes into account the way our world is constructed would almost guarantee that you will not always be on time for an appointment. Second, nothing horrible or terrible or life-threatening will occur if one is late for an appointment. It isn't likely that the person with whom you have the appointment will be totally rejecting. There is simply nothing life-threatening about being late.

In the case of my patient, the worst possible outcome is that she would have lost some therapeutic time which could have easily been made up in the future. I was not at all upset that she was late and even if I were, that would be my faulty SAD and have little to do with the patient. We discussed these issues for some time and then developed the following treatment plan:

Twice each week my patient was purposely going to be late for an appointment and then do a reanalysis of her SADs if she felt upset or vasoconstricted. Initially, my patient found it quite difficult to be late, even though she had agreed to do so during our therapy hour. But after the first six times of being up to thirty minutes late for an appointment, she came to the conclusion that no law of nature was being violated when she was late. There was hardly any inconvenience to herself or to others when she was late. At those times when there was some moderate amount of inconvenience, it was easily compensated for in the future.

I suggest that if you are one of those unfortunate enough to be so concerned about being on time that you produce vasoconstrictions for yourself, you begin a systematic program of purposely being late several times each week and reanalyze any SADs that occur. Continue being late and reanalyzing SADs until you are perfectly comfortable with this very natural state of affairs.

An important use of assertion

I'm going to end this chapter with what is, perhaps, the most important use of assertion in terms of controlling your migraine pain. Throughout this book, I have made many specific suggestions: biofeedback, Medlax exercises, SAD reanalyses, and assertiveness on a regular basis. Unfortunately, most of my patients at one time or another fall behind in practicing their vasodilation skills. The typical reason that they give for not following my suggestions on a regular basis is that someone else's demands on their time did not allow them to take even four minutes to do a biofeedback attempt or two minutes to do a Medlax. You probably have already experienced this problem. You have had difficulty in asserting your right to spend some time just for yourself.

I'm going to make a very strong statement right now, which perhaps will be offensive to some readers of this book. *You are the most important person in the world.* Your health and comfort are first and foremost. You are entitled to take the time to do biofeedback attempts and Medlaxing and whatever else it is that will make you feel better. I know this sounds selfish, but there is really something very paradoxical about being selfish in this way. If you really think you are the most important person in the world and, in fact, go ahead and do the various exercises that I have suggested to you, you will find that you really can do more for others around you.

By not asserting yourself and your importance, you perhaps can momentarily think that you are being unselfish, but sooner or later you will be in extreme pain and misery which places you in the position of not only being unable to help yourself but also being unable to help others. If you don't take care of yourself, you can't help others. Be good to yourself, take care of your arteries, and then perhaps you will have time to be good to everyone else.

You are the most important person in the world. Your health and comfort are first and foremost.

Now that you have read this far—

Now that you have read this far, I will briefly review the suggestions that I have made to help you eliminate or reduce your migraine pain.

1. Using the biotic band, try to raise your finger temperature as much as possible within a three- to four-minute period at least three to four times each day. Remember to say "vasodi-

late" to yourself before each attempt at biofeedback, as well as before each Medlax practice.

2. In order to improve your awareness of finger temperature (and vasoconstrictions), guess what your finger temperature is before you read the biotic band.

3. Practice the Medlax at least every other hour during your waking day.

4. When you notice that a vasoconstriction has occurred or that you have become emotionally upset, first say the word "vaso-dilate" to yourself and briefly attempt to use whatever vaso-dilation skills you have to stop and reverse the vasoconstriction. Second, look for and reanalyze the SAD.

5. Consider yourself to be an important person who has the right to state your feelings and assert yourself. Use the word *no*.

7

OFFENSIVE
MIGRAINE CONTROL

The best defense is a good offense. This is an adage often heard in the world of sports. Rather than waiting for the world to act on you and then taking some defensive maneuver to avoid unpleasant consequences, use the skills in this book to take the offensive and fight those conditions that produce a migraine headache. Taking the offensive is the same as using the preventive approach. Whether you think you need it or not, it is a good idea regularly to vasodilate during the day as an extra protection against unexpected and unforeseen events that may produce a vasoconstriction.

Let's say that you have met a great many SADs during the day and you have not reanalyzed these SADs or used your vasodilation skills to counteract the vasoconstrictions. Your arteries might then be relatively vasoconstricted, but not to the point where you feel uncomfortable or stressed. They may not even be vasoconstricted to the point where this particular mild level would produce a migraine headache. All of us can stand a certain amount of vasoconstriction as long as it's not too great. Unexpectedly, let's say you then get a call from Johnny's teacher, who tells you that she is extremely concerned about his mental abilities and doesn't think that he should be passed on to the third grade with the other children. SAD. Bang! More vasoconstriction occurs in your body and is added to the mild vasoconstriction already present before the telephone rang. The two have combined now to set you on an inevitable course leading to migraine pain.

If your vasodilation skills are strong enough and if you have the presence of mind to remember to use them, perhaps you actually can avoid a migraine at this point by gently opening your arteries and doing a reanalysis of your SAD to prove to yourself that the telephone call is really not a threat to life or a violation of a law of nature. The job would be even easier, however, if you had been regularly practicing vasodilation during the day prior to the teacher's phone call. The moderate amount of initial vasoconstriction would then not have been present at the time of the telephone call. Your reaction to the SAD would not have resulted in as large an amount of vasoconstriction. The chances that your vasodilation and reanalysis skills could get you off the road to migraine would be greatly enhanced.

Regularly practicing vasodilation during the day will give you a protective shield that will greatly improve your ability to reverse vasoconstrictions that come from unexpected sources. For this reason I consider regular practice of vasodilation to be an offensive move that leads to maximum prevention and protection.

What to do during the pain phase

All of the techniques in this book are aimed at allowing you to prevent the occurrence of migraine headaches. If these techniques are truly appropriate for you and are applied in the way that I have suggested, then the headache will be prevented. These techniques may not always, however, be the one hundred percent perfectly appropriate ones for you. Further, you may not always apply them in the ways that I have suggested. Hence, all of your headaches may not be prevented. Even if you can't prevent every headache, the few that you do have may be greatly reduced in intensity or duration. At times the headache may still occur in its full-blown, severe form. Although many of the techniques that I have discussed can be helpful for some patients during the pain of a migraine headache, it is usually difficult to modify bodily reactions during this phase of the headache. Once things have reached this state of affairs, you either have to lie down and go to sleep, see your doctor for pain-relieving medication and/or try the muscle relaxation and imagery techniques described below.

The relaxation of these head, face, and shoulder muscles and the imagery technique given below are the only techniques given in this book that I suggest patients use to reduce pain once the headache starts. I have purposely underemphasized techniques that can be used to reduce pain since it clearly puts the cart before the horse. What we have been seeking in the treatment plan given in this book is the prevention and eventual elimination of the headache itself.

Muscle relaxation technique for symptomatic
treatment of migraine headache pain

The technique described below and the one that follows are specifically presented to you so that you can reduce or terminate the pain after your headache has started. However, I cannot emphasize

The best way to treat migraine headaches is to prevent them from occurring in the first place.

enough the notion that the best way to treat migraine headaches is to prevent them from occurring in the first place. I am, therefore, somewhat reluctant to talk about symptomatic treatment of the pain that occurs once the headache has taken place. I describe these symptomatic treatment techniques because they have been helpful to many of my patients, but, I must caution you once more, these symptomatic treatments are not a substitute for stopping vasoconstrictions and preventing the headaches from occurring in the first place.

The muscle relaxation technique is based on the following observation: When migraine pain starts, the body naturally reacts by tensing muscles, particularly those in the shoulders, neck, head, and face. It is perfectly natural for you to react in this way because the pain is clearly a tiger with the sounds and stripes of a life-threatening event. As I pointed out earlier, you probably already have excessive muscle tension in those areas even before the pain starts. In fact, this excessive muscle tension may have been wholly or partially responsible for the vasoconstrictions which produced the headache itself.

When the migraine pain hits, you are probably adding additional muscle tension due to your reflexive response to the pain. For many patients, the prolonged pain that occurs with a migraine headache is probably due more to these tense muscles than to the dilated arteries. As migraine sufferers are well aware, the location and type of pain that you experience during a headache goes through several phases. Many of my patients report that during the latter phase of the headache, the pain becomes less pulsating or throbbing and more of a steady dull sensation. Further, after the pain itself has gone away, some patients report tenderness in the neck, shoulder, and other areas of the head or face as though their muscles had been strained and become sensitive.

These findings indicate that muscle tension not only plays a causative role in producing the headache itself but also may be a reaction to the headache, which in turn further exacerbates or worsens the experience. Thus, learning how to relax head, face, and shoulder muscles not only can be helpful in preventing headaches (in doing the Medlax, attention was paid to these muscles), but also can help you reduce the amount of pain once the headache itself starts.

I would like to anticipate some confusion that might arise from the fact that earlier in this book I suggested that you use muscle relaxation to dilate your arteries to counteract vasoconstrictions and thus avoid migraine headaches. In this section, I am also advising that you relax muscles even though you might be in the pain phase of a headache and arteries would be dilated already. That is, the same technique which is used to prevent headaches by causing vasodilation is also being used during the pain phase of the headache in which vasodilation is present. I think it can be reasonably asked,

"Wouldn't this make the headache pain worse?"

Once the pain phase of the headache begins, the rules of the game change. Your reaction to a tiger when you are in the pain phase is not going to be the same set of physiological responses that you would find when you are not having a migraine headache. For example, many patients will report very cold hands during the pain phase of the migraine headache. This would seem to be in contradiction to the notion I have been presenting that vasodilation occurs during pain. Although I have discussed this seeming contradiction earlier in the book, I think it needs further emphasis at this time.

Cold hands, cold head. That when there's a vasoconstriction in your fingers, a vasoconstriction also occurs in your head, is true only during the preheadache phase of a migraine. Thus the biotic band is a useful indicator of vasodilation and vasoconstriction in your head only during the prepain phase. It is not a good indicator of what is going on with the arteries in your head during the pain phase of the headache. It is, therefore, very possible for some people to show decreased fingertip temperature during a migraine attack whereas other people might show an increase in fingertip temperature during the very same phase of the headache.

I have found that for some patients a muscle relaxation exercise during the pain phase is helpful, whereas for others, although rather rare, it has actually increased the pain experience. If you are one of these latter individuals, then, of course, do not use the muscle relaxation technique described in this section for dealing with your headache pain. If, however, you find that the muscle relaxation technique does not increase your pain experience, then I would advise you to use it during the headache since it could very well help reduce some of the unpleasant and painful aftereffects of a headache.

Here are the muscles that I would like you to relax regularly, that is every ten minutes or so during the pain phase of your headache. The first is the frontalis muscle, the muscle in and above your forehead. If you place your fingers on your forehead and raise your eyebrows as if in surprise, you will feel your forehead wrinkle and the frontalis muscle contract. Hold your frontalis muscle in a contracted position for about the count of ten seconds while leaving your hand in position on your forehead. Now tell yourself the word "release" and let the frontalis muscle relax and allow your forehead to smooth out as much as possible. Once this has occurred try to let the muscle relax even more. If you notice it starting to tighten again, try to let it relax.

The next muscle I would like you to learn how to relax is the jaw, or masseter, muscle. Hold your head in an erect position and grasp your lower jaw around the chin with the thumb and forefinger, with the thumb below the chin and the forefinger above. Now rapidly try to move your lower jaw up and down with your hand. If you feel resistance, then your jaw muscle is not relaxed. Allow your jaw to relax and repeat the experiment until you can rapidly move your jaw up and down with your hand without voluntarily using the jaw muscles. Be careful you don't bite your tongue while doing this particular muscle relaxation exercise. Remember, if you cannot move your jaw rapidly up and down, it means that your jaw muscle is tense and holding the jaw in a rigid position. Similarly if you find that your whole head moves when you attempt to move just your lower jaw, it again means that the masseter muscle is very tense.

Next I would like you to learn how to relax the neck muscle. The neck muscle is actually a complex set of muscles that allow you to move the head around and back and forth. Try to find a position where your head is balanced on your shoulders just as a teeter-totter is perfectly balanced when two people of equal weight are equidistant from the center point. Your neck is completely relaxed when a slight movement of your head in any direction from this point of perfect balance will result in your head just flopping over in that direction. If you move your head just slightly forward from this balanced position, it will flop over just like a rag doll's head would if, when perfectly balanced upright, a small amount of forward pressure were applied.

To summarize, these are the three muscles that I would like you to pay particular attention to: the forehead, or frontalis; the jaw, or masseter; and the neck. During the pain phase of a headache, it is advisable to check the muscles every ten minutes until you are so aware of these muscles that you automatically make sure they are relaxed as much as possible. Hopefully, the relaxation of these muscles will help to reduce not only the pain of your migraine attack but also some of the lingering aftereffects. Let us now proceed with the next technique that can be used during the pain of a migraine headache.

Imagery technique for dealing with the pain of migraine headache

Many of my patients have found helpful one additional technique in dealing with their headaches once the pain phase has begun: "Imagery" may be used to reduce and even eliminate the pain.

To begin with, please don't ask me why this particular technique actually reduces pain because I don't have a good answer. I'm actually somewhat at a loss to explain how or why the technique works when it does. It's one of those things that just seems to work for some people some of the time, and I include it for that reason.

After you are first aware that the pain phase of your headache has begun, sit back in a comfortable chair and close your eyes. Very briefly attempt to relax your entire body if at all possible. Now relax the three muscles described previously. I realize there may be extreme pain at this point and any attempt at relaxation might be very difficult, and if you are now in the pain phase of a headache, you probably have very little hope or motivation to engage in either this or the muscle relaxation technique. So, I'm not asking you to have faith or an expectation that this technique is going to help. I'm just going to ask you to try doing it and whatever will happen will happen.

All right, you're sitting back in your chair, your eyes are closed, you have attempted to relax your body. Now I want you to imagine in your mind's eye the color, shape, sound, and odor of your headache. Start with one of these characteristcs first and then add the others one by one as the image begins to gain clarity. For example, let us say you begin with color. What color comes to mind when you conjure up the image of your headache in your mind's eye? Now, once you have the color, what kind of shape does your headache have? I'd like to point out that it may not have any shape or its shape may be changing, but, in any event, whatever happens at this point is just fine. Next, does your headache have a sound? If so, try to imagine it and allow it to have a clarity also. Finally, what odor comes to mind? If none does, that's perfectly fine, if one does, then it will simply add to the complexity of the image.

Now that you have considered each of these four characteristics in your image of your headache, continue to concentrate on this image. As you do, one or more of these characteristics may change. When this happens, just allow it to happen and observe it as if you were watching a motion picture projected on a screen in front of you. Continue with this process for five to ten minutes noting the change in shape, color, sound, and odor as you do so. Most of my patients find this technique to be helpful in reducing the pain of their headaches. If you have gone through this process and you are one of those fortunate enough to benefit from it, then continue to use the process as frequently as you would like to give yourself some relief.

If it did not work for you the first time you tried it, do not despair. I have found that it can still be of benefit to individuals who had no success on their initial try. Try it again, perhaps a half-hour after your initial attempt, and see if you can make any progress. If you've tried the technique several times, and it has not produced any relief, then you know you are one of those for whom this will not be of benefit.

If you are one of those for whom the technique has been helpful, please remember that this or the muscle relaxation technique is not to be used as a substitute for following all of the other procedures and techniques described in this book. The best long-term solution for eliminating your headaches really will come from dealing with the initial nonpain phase or vasoconstrictive phase of your headache. Of course, there is no harm in using the imagery technique, and I think one should feel fortunate if it does produce relief from pain. Just remember to keep up your Medlax and analysis of SADs, as well as using the other procedures previously discussed in order to eliminate those headaches once and for all.

Incidentally, if you are one of those patients for whom lying down makes things worse, do not be alarmed. Many migraine sufferers find that lying down or resting actually tends to increase the throbbing pain that they experience. From my point of view, I believe this indicates that relaxing during this phase of the headache may actually produce a small increase in vasodilation and hence pain. I have great empathy for migraine sufferers, in general, and in particular for those whose pain seems to be made worse by almost anything that they try to do.

Prevention is really the answer

It is unfortunate that I do not have good advice for what can be done once the pain starts other than not reacting to the headache with the Analysis "I should not be having this headache." I discussed this particular SAD in chapter 5 and pointed out that it can only make an already painful situation even worse. It is fortunate, however, that a great deal of the pain and discomfort of a migraine can be avoided by doing something before the painful vasodilation.

The emphasis then is on prevention. The emphasis then is on prevention. That is why I have paid so much attention to the nonpainful vasoconstriction which is the precursor of your migraine headache. During the vasoconstriction you can effectively intervene and change these initial reactions which often lead to a migraine. I have often been asked, "Does every vasoconstriction lead to a migraine headache?" The chances are that only a fraction of the vasoconstrictions lead to a migraine headache, but it is difficult to tell which will lead to a migraine and which will not. A single vasoconstriction may not lead to a headache, although if another occurs within a short period of time after the first, there may be an accumulated effect. One single vasoconstriction may not produce a migraine headache but each one may very well play its part in the eventual onset of the headache itself. As I pointed out earlier, once you have vasoconstricted, even if only to a small degree, you then become more vulnerable to future vasoconstrictions.

Therefore, our general plan is to stop as many vasoconstrictions as possible. Stopping these vasoconstrictions is going to be of benefit even though you may stop many that would not have produced a migraine in the first place. Remember that a vasoconstriction is a reaction to danger signals on the part of your body. It places stresses and strains on almost every system ranging from your heart, liver, and lungs to perhaps even the immune system in your blood, which, over time, could lead to other medical problems.

The recent emphasis on managing stress in one's life in order to stop crippling disorders such as heart attack, hypertension, stroke, stomach problems, etc., is directly related to the kinds of reactions you have that lead to migraine headaches. I am not saying that you are more prone to get other medical problems, it's just that you have a symptom, headache, which makes you more aware of stress than other people. So even though you may be preventing vasoconstrictions which wouldn't have led to a migraine headache, you are going to receive benefits in terms of how you will feel, think, and perhaps avoid other medical problems in the long term.

How long before your headaches go away?

I have delayed attempting to answer this question because I believe that you are probably in a better position to answer it than I am. Hopefully, you have been reading this book regularly and practicing the various techniques that I have suggested. Hopefully, you have also noticed a decrease or perhaps elimination of your headaches by this time. You can use your experience with reduction of headache pain to make a prediction as to how long it will take before your headaches improve or are eliminated altogether.

Some of my patients become disappointed when they find that they are unable to use the biofeedback experience to raise their finger temperature or to vasodilate. Keep in mind that people respond differently to the biofeedback training experience. Some of them learn very quickly in several days of practice. Others may take weeks or even months before they have finally developed the skill of raising their hand temperature by dilating arteries that supply blood to the limbs. Some people can never learn how to do this.

The cause of these differences is not understood. It used to be thought that only young individuals could learn how to control bodily functions through biofeedback. I have had many senior citizens as patients, however, who have done a splendid job of learning to control their physiology. Whether or not you learn how to control handwarming depends on how right this particular technique is for you, how diligently you practice, what your lifelong experiences have been in tuning in to your body, etc.

If you do not progress quickly or never learn how to warm your hands through these techniques it is not a reflection on you and you should not blame yourself. It also does not mean that this book is of no use to you because you will find that two-thirds of this book is devoted to techniques having very little to do with warming one's hands through biofeedback and instead suggests other methods to combat vasoconstrictions. These other techniques, such as the Medlax and reanalysis of SADs, as well as the dietary approach given in chapter 8, can be sufficient to greatly reduce or stop migraine headaches. My advice to those of you who have difficulty with hand warming is, first of all, don't give it up, try it every now and then to see if you may stumble on or discover a way of doing it. Second, proceed with the rest of the techniques and use these wherever they are applicable. You only stand to benefit from this strategy.

8

FOOD AND MIGRAINE

Still having headaches?

If you have read the previous chapters and have been regularly following my suggestions and you are still having headaches, then this chapter is for you. Although you might be convinced that your headaches are not caused by foods, if you have not yet adequately controlled your migraines, it is extremely important that you read this chapter. There is reason to believe that using the techniques you already know in combination with the additional techniques given in this chapter will be very effective. Or if you have tried to control your headaches through dietary means and were not successful, this chapter should be read in detail. My answer to the mystery of the relationship between food and migraines will explain why you may have been unsuccessful in attempting to eliminate your headaches through dietary means—and how you can now be successful.

How food can be related to migraines

There are many different ways that your arteries can become constricted. It is important that you be aware of all these sources of vasoconstriction so that you can maximally combat them to prevent headaches. The prevention of a vasoconstriction can make you less vulnerable to an eventual migraine headache. Keep in mind that the techniques that you have been learning thus far are aimed at preventing vasoconstrictions and/or producing vasodilations. When you analyze SADs, you are stopping the outside world from interfering with your blood flow. When you regularly do the Medlax you are making sure that there is sufficient vasodilation so that even if an emergency arises, you will not get a headache. The use of biofeedback and the biotic band allows you to detect when a vasoconstriction has occurred and then directly combat it by gently dilating arteries and preventing the sequence that leads to head pain. Hopefully you're regularly practicing the skills aimed at neutralizing these various sources of vasoconstriction.

There is, however, one more source of vasoconstriction that should be considered by many migraine sufferers. This is the food that you eat. I would like to emphasize, however, that not all migraine sufferers react to foods. Furthermore, of those who do—not all react in the same way. In fact, it is most likely that you react to only *one* of the three ways that food might bring on migraine.

There are three primary ways in which the foods you eat can cause vasoconstrictions and hence make you vulnerable to a headache.

There are three primary ways in which the foods you eat can cause vasoconstrictions and hence make you vulnerable to a headache:

1. The food may actually contain a substance that directly affects your arteries and hence produces a vasoconstriction. Coffee with its caffeine is well known for this effect. There are many other foods, however, containing substances that can have a similar action on your arteries. I will discuss these foods a little bit later under the heading of "chemical reactions."

Food may contain a substance that directly affects your arteries.

2. The food can affect your arteries through an allergic reaction. Allergic reactions to food are very complex, but there is reason to believe that one effect of an allergy response is a vasoconstriction of arteries supplying blood to your brain.

Foods might cause an allergic reaction.

3. The food can bring about migraines through nutritional and functional deficiencies—and in particular the low blood sugar syndrome called hypoglycemia, which will be explained and discussed later.

Migraine might be caused by hypoglycemia.

It is important for you to avoid this troublesome source of vasoconstriction regardless of whether it is from direct chemical stimulation (such as caffeine) or an allergic response or low blood sugar. I will discuss how to determine which of these three might be important to your migraine prevention program.

A migraine headache is brought on by several sources of vasoconstriction that occur in the same period of time.

Keep in mind that the whole approach in this book is based on the fact that there are many sources of vasoconstrictions other than foods and at times any one of those sources may produce a strong enough vasoconstriction over a long enough period of time that it will eventually lead to a vasodilation and painful migraine headache. It is more likely however, that a migraine headache is brought on by several sources of vasoconstriction which occur by chance at the same time. For example, a certain amount of vasoconstriction is caused by drinking several cups of coffee during the day. If you have been drinking coffee during the day and then come home to be confronted by a SAD, such as the water pipes have frozen and burst in your home and you do not have sufficient money to remedy the damage, the combination of events—the coffee and the frozen water

It's important to consider all the sources of vasoconstriction, only one of which may be dietary.

pipes—might be sufficient to produce a headache. If you had prevented vasoconstrictions from either of these two sources, you may not have suffered the migraine: if you had reanalyzed the SADs concerning your pipes or if you had not drunk the coffee or if you had regularly practiced Medlax during the day. It's important to consider all the sources of vasoconstriction, only one of which may be dietary. For that reason I would like you to consider the foods you eat as possible sources of vasoconstriction, which can combine in the manner described above to produce a headache.

Is this chapter for you?

Those of you who know your headaches are brought on by certain foods would have eliminated them by now and probably would not be suffering from migraines. The vast majority of migraine sufferers however, do not associate their headaches with a particular kind of food. One of the first reactions that you may have had to the idea that foods are related to migraines is that, in your experience, this simply is not true! You have not been able to associate your headaches with any particular food that you have eaten. You may even have been suspicious of certain foods but then concluded that your suspicion was unfounded. For example, you may have thought that eating oranges in some way was related to your headaches. You may have then stopped eating oranges and you still had headaches. Similarly, at other times you may have noted that even though you ate oranges, you did not get a migraine. This chapter is for individuals who feel that foods are not related to the occurrence of their migraine headaches because nothing could be further from the truth.

> **This chapter is for individuals who feel that foods are not related to the occurrence of their migraine headaches.**

It is possible for foods to play a role in your migraine headaches and for you not to be aware of a reaction to foods that is a precondition for head pain. In order to better explain why you may have a hidden reaction to foods which, in turn, contributes to your migraines, I'm going to discuss a mystery concerning food and migraines.

> **It is possible for foods to play a role in your migraine headaches and you would not be aware of it.**

Food and migraine: A mystery is solved

In my study of migraine headaches, I did a "review of the literature." I read hundreds of articles written during the past one hundred years on the causes and cures of migraine headaches. I naturally put more faith in the most recent articles since they are based on knowledge accumulated over the years, and they use the latest technology and methods of data collection. From a historical perspective—if I look at trends through the years—a very curious and interesting mystery has appeared: the role of diet and food allergies in the treatment of migraines. The fact that eating certain foods can bring on headaches has long been recognized in the medical literature. It was, however, seen as a relatively unimportant factor until the late 1950s and early 1960s.

At that point there suddenly was a blossoming of interest in food allergies and an accumulation of evidence that related diet and allergic reactions to migraines. One scientist went so far as to state quite boldly that "all migraines were caused by allergic reactions." Innumerable case histories were given in which individuals who suffered from migraine headaches and were treated to no avail by every known method were able to completely eliminate their headaches by not eating certain foods, such as eggs, milk, or pork. However, enthusiasm began to wane in the years following this heyday of dietary factors in migraines. Gradually throughout the years, the role of diet as a cause of migraine headaches was written about less and less until finally, in today's literature on migraines, it may not even be mentioned.

Why did so many doctors at one time believe that eating certain kinds of foods caused migraine headaches, whereas at a later time they considered these same dietary factors to be relatively unimportant? Well, the answer is straightforward.

Some people were able to eliminate their headaches by avoiding certain foods in their diets. However, the vast majority of patients followed their doctor's orders and diligently eliminated certain foods from their diet but were not helped and continued to suffer from their headaches. So, although the doctors were encouraged by the fact that a few of their patients got better, the number of patients who improved was too small to consider dietary factors as being very important. The nagging question that remains is, Why were some people (although few in number) and not others helped by controlling dietary factors? I will attempt to answer this question a little later in this chapter and show you why dietary factors are important for many more patients than is currently believed. First, I would like to discuss some perplexing scientific findings about certain foods and migraine headaches and another part of the mystery that needs to be solved.

Dietary migraines

A survey was made of a large number of migraine sufferers to discover if they believe that certain foods do tend to bring on the headache. A substantial number of patients state that certain foods do precipitate or tend to bring on attacks. I refer to such patients as "dietary migraine patients." If you then ask these patients what foods in particular tend to bring on the attack, certain foods are mentioned more often than others.

FOOD	PERCENTAGE
Chocolate and cola	74
Dairy products, including milk	46
Citrus fruits	30
Eggs	25
Alcohol	25
Fatty fried foods	18
Onions	17
Pork	14
Coffee	14
Seafood	10

One researcher in England made an interesting observation while going over this and similar lists obtained in other studies: Many (but not all) of these foods contain a natural chemical substance called tyramine (pronounced like tear-a-mean), a substance that is known to directly affect the opening and closing of arteries and easily could be a direct cause of migraine headaches. Please do not start any diets yet—complete this chapter before you attempt any dietary treatment. While many of the foods in the "most wanted list" contain tyramine, many of the suspect foods definitely do not. But, it seems possible that tyramine might be implicated, at least for some dietary migraines.

The conclusions that can be drawn from this work on tyramine have applications to food allergy reactions, as well as hypoglycemic reactions.

Further experiments were done, which I'm going to discuss in some detail since they are both interesting and important to our understanding of the role of tyramine (as well as other dietary factors) in migraine headaches. More importantly, this tyramine research has implications for understanding how foods *in general* can relate to headaches and have application to food allergy reactions as well as hypoglycemic reactions.

Research on tyramine

The English scientist Dr. Edda Hanington, who first noted that tyramine seemed to be present in many of the foods that dietary migrainers reported, performed a very interesting experiment. Migraine headache patients were asked to volunteer for an experiment in which they would be asked to swallow a capsule containing an experimental substance. Each of the volunteers then received in the mail an envelope containing an unmarked capsule. Half of the patients received a capsule containing pure tyramine, the other half received a capsule with an inert substance (a placebo). They were then asked to record whether or not they got a headache in the twenty-four hours following ingestion of the capsule. Sure enough, by the end of the day, those patients who had taken the tyramine had severe migraine attacks, whereas those who had taken the placebo experienced no such pain. This same experiment was duplicated time and time again and seemed to show conclusively that the ingestion of tyramine is likely to bring on an attack in dietary migraine patients. However, there is an interesting and curious mystery about the role of tyramine in headaches.

The same experiment was done again in the United States by an American doctor. In this second experiment, there was no difference in results between those who took tyramine and those who took the placebo. Neither produced a large number of migraine headaches. Perplexed, this American scientist repeated the experiment again, but this time with a larger dose of tyramine, exceeding even those doses given by the doctor in England. Once again, the tyramine did not produce migraine headaches. At the same time that the American experiments were being conducted and producing no migraine headaches, the English experiments were continued, and the tyramine did produce migraine headaches. Hence, the mystery. Why does tyramine in the English experiments produce migraine headaches while tyramine in the American experiments does not? I want to give you one more important finding from an experiment, and then I'll give you my theory to explain these contradictory results.

In an experiment performed by a third researcher, dietary migraine subjects were brought into the laboratory. The third researcher was under the impression that tyramine would always bring about headaches in such patients since he was not aware of the contradictory American findings. The purpose of the experiment was not to test whether tyramine would bring on a headache, but assuming that the chemical would bring on a headache at a known time and place (i.e., in the laboratory after taking tyramine), further studies could then be done on changes in the brain—as measured by an EEG— during a migraine attack. That is, this third scientist was really interested in measuring the brain waves that accompany a migraine headache. Normally, this could only be done through circumstance and luck: The patient would have to be in the doctor's laboratory at the onset of a migraine headache. Since migraines are sporadic and unpredictable, this occurred very infrequently. However, after reading the English doctor's results, Doctor Number Three felt that if tyramine could be given to patients and headaches were likely to occur, then his important research could be conducted.

The patients all faithfully reported to his laboratory, and he gave them doses of tyramine. He then connected them to his brain wave machinery and waited for headaches to appear. The results of tyramine ingestion in Doctor Three's lab were similar to the American doctor's results. Very few people got migraine headaches. However, nearly all of these dietary migraine sufferers showed abnormal brain wave activity after eating tyramine. So, although tyramine did not evoke a migraine headache, it did affect these patients by producing some small changes in brain waves. However, the effects of the tyramine were harmless and could only be detected on the brain wave equipment. The patients reported no discomfort, pain, aura, or anything else. In fact, if the brain wave equipment had not been attached to these subjects, there would have been no way of knowing that the tyramine produced any effects whatsoever (unless they were wearing a biotic band, of course!).

A solution to the mystery

Now we have three facts which go into making up the mystery: An English doctor found that tyramine produces migraine headaches in dietary migraine patients; an American doctor found that tyramine does not produce migraine headaches; a third doctor found that tyramine does not produce headaches or other symptoms but does produce changes in brain wave activity. My theory is that tyramine *by itself* is not sufficient to produce headaches in certain dietary migraine patients. However, when tyramine is ingested and combines with other sources of vasoconstriction (e.g., a danger signal), a headache will result.

According to this theory, in the experiment conducted by the English doctor, it was found that tyramine produced headaches because her patients took their pills at home and went about their usual activities (work, school, child care, etc.). These usual activities produced the usual stress that we encounter on a day-to-day basis and this stress probably produced a certain amount of vasoconstriction. These patients can be contrasted with those in the other two experiments who did not get as many headaches and were removed from their usual sources of stress, SAD's, etc., because they spent the day in a laboratory or clinic rather than at home or work. In other words, the English doctor's subjects were vasoconstricted because they reacted to the usual SAD's confronted on a day-to-day basis. This then combined with the vasoconstriction produced by food, and the patients developed a migraine. The fact that tyramine alone produces a reaction not sufficient enough to cause a migraine but sufficient enough to be detectable with very sensitive recording equipment attached to the subject's head was shown by the third researcher.

So, my theory is that certain foods and other dietary factors all by themselves may at times produce migraines in certain people. However, I believe that migraine headaches are caused more often by these foods when combined with other sources of vasoconstriction, such as danger signals, or if the patient's overconstricted arteries have not been vasodilated through the use of the Medlax and/or biofeedback. Diet, by itself, is not enough to prevent migraines.

Diet by itself is not enough to prevent migraines.

The most important sources of migraine headaches, in my experience, have been discussed in the previous chapters of this book. In fact, many migraine sufferers can eliminate their pain solely by following the procedures previously outlined and ignore dietary factors.

However, if you have followed the instructions this far and still

It is the *combination* of a food reaction with vasoconstricted arteries that sets the stage for a migraine.

In order to stop your migraines, it is necessary to vasodilate regularly and eliminate certain foods from your diet.

feel you have room for more improvement, then I would suggest using the techniques outlined (Medlax, biofeedback, assertiveness, etc.) in combination with the dietary recommendations in this chapter. Those individuals who may have tried to control their headaches through diet may have been unsuccessful because they did not have the necessary vasodilation techniques discussed earlier in this book. I would strongly urge you to follow your dietary regimen once again, only this time regularly practice vasodilation skills at the same time. Remember, it is the *combination* of a food reaction with vasoconstricted arteries that sets the stage for a migraine. In order to stop your migraines it is necessary to vasodilate regularly *and* eliminate certain foods from your diet or correct for other dietary problems as discussed below.

Before you rush off and attempt to eliminate foods with tyramine in them (I'll have more to say about this later), keep in mind that the above obtained results were for those individuals who thought that certain foods did produce migraine headaches. Even if food does play a role in a patient's migraine, most people would not suspect the food because, in my theory, a food reaction is usually not sufficient by itself to produce a headache. The food reaction must occur in combination to cause a headache. Given my theory that it requires a combination of a food reaction plus vasoconstriction to produce a headache, a great multitude of migraine sufferers (even those with no suspicion of food reaction) can benefit from controlling their food consumption. As you will see, I do have some advice on how to discover which, if any, dietary factors might play a role in your headaches.

Resistance and delayed reactions

The concepts of delayed reaction times and resistance can obscure dietary triggers for most migraine headache sufferers. It is important that you be familiar with these concepts before you reject the notion that your own headaches, in fact, might be produced by some of the foods you eat.

Resistance

The concept of resistance is important in understanding the relationship between some of the foods you eat and the occurrence of a migraine headache. The term *resistance* means that after you experience a headache, your body produces a natural reaction that prevents you from getting additional headaches produced by the same food for a certain period of time. The mechanism underlying resistance is not well understood, but the fact that resistance does occur is well established. If you are fortunate, the resistance period is long enough so that you can regularly eat one of these foods and perhaps not experience a disrupting rate of headaches. Some individuals, however, may have resistance periods of only an hour or so; therefore, they may experience a headache triggered by certain foods on a very regular basis. This natural delayed response can often mask or hide a potential food trigger eaten on a regular basis.

Let's say for example, that eggs trigger migraine headaches for you and you eat eggs four or five times a week. You would then expect to have four or five migraine headaches a week, but instead—due to resistance—you might only experience a headache every two weeks or every three weeks. Thus, you can see that if you were reactive to eggs and resistant to the effects of eggs for two to three weeks after you had a headache, it would be very difficult for you to discover the relationship between eggs and headaches. You would never even suspect that eggs were a trigger. It is this phenomenon of resistance more than any other factor that is perhaps responsible for migraine headache sufferers not discovering dietary triggers for their pain.

Delayed Reactions

Human beings seem to vary in almost every characteristic. We all speak differently, we all look different, and we all have different and unique physiologic reactions. One of these differences that might contribute to your not being aware of the relationship between foods you eat and your headaches could be the long delayed reaction period. Let's get back to our egg example. If there were a fourteen- to thirty-two-hour delay between the time that you eat the eggs and the time that you experience symptoms, you can see the difficulty in identifying eggs as a trigger.

Even if food does play a role in a patient's migraine, most people would not suspect because (my theory) a food reaction by itself is usually not sufficient to produce a headache. The food reaction must occur in combination with vasoconstriction to produce a headache. Nevertheless, many migraine sufferers (even those with no suspicion of food reaction) can benefit from controlling their food intake. Later I will offer some advice on how to find out which, if any, dietary factors play a role in your headaches.

Allergic reactions

Up to this point, I have focused primarily on the role of tyramine in producing migraine headaches. There are two other important ways that foods can be related to headaches. I would now like to discuss the allergic reaction. Some of us are probably born with a particular sensitivity to certain foods. This sensitivity is called allergy.

Recently, an article entitled "Food Allergy and Migraine" was published in *The Lancet*, a prestigious British medical journal. The doctors who wrote this article point out that migraine affects about 20 percent of the population. Using a new medical testing procedure called radioallergiosorbent (RAST) test, considered a relatively sensitive test for detecting food allergies, the doctors were able to measure the response in the blood to foods that were eaten. The study involved thirty-three patients over a two-year period. Among the foods used in the RAST test were: milk, cheese, eggs, chocolate, coffee, tea. Seventy percent of the patients tested showed an allergic response. When these same patients eliminated the above foods, in most cases they also experienced complete relief from migraine headache, usually within two weeks.

The authors of "Food Allergy and Migraine" conclude that food allergy is a very important factor in migraine headaches. The results of the RAST study indicating the importance of the allergy are striking indeed.

Fifteen to twenty years ago most doctors thought that food allergies were extremely important in migraine headaches. At the present time, the role of food allergy as well as other dietary factors are (erroneously—in my opinion) viewed as less important. My theory is that those doctors who attempted to treat migraine headaches by having their patients eliminate foods to which they were allergic did not go far enough. The doctors were not aware that it required both the allergic reaction and vasoconstriction from other sources to produce the headache itself. Since diet only eliminated one source of vasoconstriction, this treatment was largely unsuccessful.

I recently had an opportunity to explore this hypothesis with a patient, a young woman, twenty-one years of age, who had been suffering from severe migraine headaches for over six years. She would have one or two headaches every week and end up in the emergency room receiving pain-killing injections several times each year. When she first got these migraine headaches, her parents suggested to their family doctor that allergy might be playing a role since they both suffered from allergic skin reactions, and allergies often run in families. The doctor then referred his patient to an allergist who did what is called the "scratch test" in which the physician actually tests a person's skin response to a small amount of the food substance. If the patient shows an unusual amount of irritation in the form of a blister or hive, it is taken to mean that the individual is allergic to that food substance. Although this test is not without fault, a positive scratch test result might indicate an allergy to that food which in turn could play a role in causing headaches.

This particular patient had shown positive scratch test results to several foods although she showed an unusually large one to eggs. Based on this information, the physician suggested that she eliminate eggs from her diet to see if her headache frequency decreased. She faithfully followed her doctor's instructions and stopped eating eggs.

Unfortunately, she did not notice any change in her condition. She also liked eggs and felt it was a great inconvenience to no longer eat them. So, after several months, she started to eat eggs again.

In my examination of this patient, I found that she suffered considerably from vasoconstricted arteries caused by her lack of assertiveness and inability to say no as well as a lack of vasodilation skills that could have prevented some of the severe vasoconstrictions she experienced on a daily basis. My treatment program consisted of biofeedback and assertiveness training, as well as instructions in the use of the Medlax. Just through the use of these techniques alone, she was able to cut the number of headaches in half. She now was experiencing about one headache per week; but even though she increased the number of daily Medlaxing, she was unable to show any further improvement. It was at this point that I suggested she again try to eliminate eggs from her diet. She did so and totally eliminated migraine headaches. At the time of this writing it has been over six months since we terminated our treatment and she still has not had a migraine.

This case is a good illustration of my combination theory about the relationship of food and other sources of vasoconstriction to migraine headaches. This patient previously had eliminated eggs from her diet without any beneficial effect because she didn't do anything about other stresses in her environment. Finally, the necessity of using vasodilation and other skills in combination with diet in the treatment of headaches was demonstrated. Most readers of this chapter may not know (1) whether or not they are allergic to foods, (2) whether foods with tyramine could be producing responses; or (3) whether their headaches might be aggravated by hypoglycemic responses. I have developed a plan for such individuals which will be discussed after I explain the nature of hypoglycemia.

Hypoglycemia

This is the last of the three dietary factors of importance to the migraine headache sufferer. In recent years, much has been written about hypoglycemia, low blood sugar. Further, it is somewhat of a controversial topic within the medical profession. Some physicians regularly check their patients for hypoglycemia; other doctors feel that because hypoglycemia occurs so rarely it is a waste of the patient's time and money to regularly test for it. Much of the controversy concerns the standardization of laboratory tests used to diagnose hypoglycemia. Controversy notwithstanding, there is strong evidence that some migraine patients will be helped by the hypoglycemic diet, and I am including hypoglycemia as a possible dietary factor in this chapter on foods and migraine because of a recent scientific study.

Hypoglycemia means that the sugar-regulating processes in

your body have been overworked and are no longer functioning in a normal way. These regulating processes normally will keep the amount of sugar in your blood at a very consistent level regardless of when and what you might have eaten. Blood sugar is important for proper physiologic functioning and a certain amount must always be present for the body to do its job. Hypoglycemia experts feel that the large amounts of sugars ingested by most people overtax the body's sugar regulatory system and it begins to malfunction. One characteristic of hypoglycemic patients is that they become extremely hungry and irritable when they have been deprived of foods with sugar. This is quickly relieved when they eat a high sugar content food, such as candy or ice cream. This recent research showed that certain migraine patients were almost certain to be cured of their headaches if they followed a hypoglycemic diet. All of these patients showed a certain time pattern to their headaches. In addition laboratory tests done on these patients by their physicians indicated the presence or possible presence of hypoglycemia. It is entirely possible to follow a hypoglycemic diet without necessarily having these tests, and some physicians, in fact, will prescribe a hypoglycemic diet as a diagnostic measure—if the patient improves it means hypoglycemia was present.

To learn whether or not you are hypoglycemic, you, of course, must consult your physician for this diagnosis.

How to select the right diet for you

I have discussed three different types of reactions to food and their relationship to migraine: (1) chemical reactions to tyramine or other substances that directly affect arteries, (2) allergic reactions, and (3) hypoglycemic reactions. The question is, which, if any, of these diets could play a role in your headaches. I'm going to give you some recommendations to help you discover the role of diet in your headaches. Whatever dietary factors you are evaluating, it is extremely important that you follow the vasodilation procedures outlined in the previous chapters of this book. Before beginning any dietary plan, check with your doctor to make sure the diet you try meets with his/her approval.

Follow these steps:

1. If you are suspicious (even if it is a nagging, mostly unconscious suspicion) that certain foods have in the past been related to your migraine pain, then immediately eliminate these foods from your diet until you have properly evaluated whether or not they are important. I'm basing this recommendation on the fact that these vague feelings might be a clue as to whether or not you are having allergic reactions to

particular foods. If you've had some vague feeling about popcorn or onion or coffee, give yourself a real chance to find out once and for all whether or not these foods are the culprits by eliminating the food and regularly doing Medlax, biofeedback, etc. Keep in mind that even if you have already tried to eliminate these foods without any effect, diet in combination with controlling other sources of vasoconstriction is likely to be rewarding. You probably were not successful in the past because migraine headaches can come from other sources of vasoconstriction, and these must be controlled before you can truly evaluate the effect of the food.

If you have no suspicions and have no reason to eliminate any particular foods from your diet, then go on to step 2.

2. Follow Diet H if you know that you are hypoglycemic or suspect so or if your headaches tend to occur in the morning before you've eaten and/or at other times when you haven't had food. For example, let's say that you only had time to drink some orange juice for breakfast and then couldn't eat lunch. If you know that this will bring about a terrible headache in the afternoon, then you might be having a hypoglycemic-caused migraine headache. If your headaches tend to come after periods of fasting (not necessarily fasting purposely, but just due to these accidental circumstances which make it difficult to eat regularly or as much as needed) then the hypoglycemic diet is the one to try. If your headaches are time-locked to midmorning or midafternoon, this is an indication that they may be caused by a hypoglycemic reaction. If any of these descriptions fit you, then try the hypoglycemic diet.

Follow Diet H if your headaches tend to occur in the morning before you've eaten and/or at other times when you haven't had food.

3. If neither of the above seems to fit, then I suggest you either follow the low-tyramine and chemical reaction diet (Diet T, given on page 115) or the standard allergy-elimination diet (Diet A described on page 114). The low-tyramine diet involves eliminating foods that contain tyramine. The allergy-elimination diet involves elimination of the most commonly reacted-to foods. There is no reason to suggest one of these diets first as opposed to the other (Diet T vs. Diet A) unless you have some hunch that one of them may hit more of the foods you suspect. But lacking any suspicions, just flip a coin and pick one. If it is not effective, then after a fair trial, go on to the other.

Good nutrition—before you try a diet

We all learned in grade school about the necessity of having a balanced nourishing diet. It is extremely important that you keep this in mind when you attempt any of the dietary procedures outlined below. For example, if you decide to eliminate pork from your diet because you have been suspicious of it for many years, and if pork is your only source of protein, then you will not be eating a well-balanced, nourishing diet. To make sure your diet is balanced, another source of protein should be substituted. Most of us eat a wide enough variety of foods so that elimination of a few will not appreciably alter the nutritional balance. It is simply a case of using good judgment when following these or any other dietary procedures. Of course, if you are under the care of a physician for some chronic disease in which dietary factors are being regulated, then do not attempt any of the suggestions made above unless your physician concurs. In any event, I recommend that you consult with your physician before altering your diet.

Diet H—the hypoglycemic diet

As I mentioned earlier, the term *hypoglycemia* means low blood sugar. This blood sugar, by the way, is extremely important. It is the only kind of energy that the brain can use and a deficient amount of blood sugar can not only contribute to your migraine headaches but produce a variety of other symptoms ranging from depression and a lack of overall energy to extreme hyperactive high tension and anxiety. It would seem that an appropriate diet would be one that contains many sugars that quickly get into the blood stream. But there is a paradox or contradictory aspect to the hypoglycemic diet described below, one that is low in sugars and other nutrients that could enter the blood stream quickly.

Here is the explanation: In the first place our diets contain horrendously large amounts of sugars which can easily exceed 125 pounds a year. The hypoglycemic condition is brought about by the fact that the body attempts to accommodate this vastly excessive sugar intake by producing a chemical called "insulin." Eventually, the glands that produce this insulin become so overworked and stimulated that most of the time the body overcompensates and too much insulin is produced and blood sugar is too low. During those times of the day that this occurs you may experience a craving for something sweet. Eating sweets at this point will give you temporary relief because the sugars are rapidly absorbed into the body and there is an initial increase in blood sugar. Unfortunately, this only exacerbates the problem since it stimulates the body's adaptive mechanisms to deal with the sugar and within a short period of time it results in the hypoglycemic or low blood sugar state. The more sugar you eat, the more immediate relief you may feel, but the worse your overall condition becomes.

The diet I describe below eliminates sugars and other types of nutrients that tend to be quickly converted into sugar and enter the blood stream quickly. The recommended foods are absorbed much more slowly and will allow the normalization of the sugar-regulating mechanisms in your body. I would like to point out that there are vast differences from person to person in the ability to tolerate sugars. Some individuals cannot take even the smallest amounts of sugar or starches (starches are quickly absorbed sources of nutrients that turn into sugar and enter the blood stream) without producing excessive insulin. By and large the more sugar and starch you can avoid, the better off you are going to be. This is especially important during the first two weeks of your diet. After the first two weeks, your body will have begun to normalize and you can at that time slightly increase the amount of sugar or starch that you eat.

The timing of meals on this hypoglycemic diet is as important as the content, and involves eating at least six meals per day. The amount that you eat at each meal, of course, is reduced so that the total consumed is the same as if you had eaten three meals. You just eat half as much at each of these meals. Again the idea here is to avoid the sudden changes in body chemistry that result from stimulating the sugar-regulating mechanisms each time you ingest large amounts of food and then don't eat for several hours thereafter. This really taxes the insulin-producing and -regulating centers in your body. Eat frequently! Avoid sugars and starches!

Diet H—foods to be eaten

Good sources of protein are meat, poultry, all types of fish and shellfish, cheese, dairy products, and eggs. Nuts, especially eaten in their raw form, are an excellent source of protein. Only recently it has been discovered that eating a variety of nuts can supply all the required proteins heretofore thought to be available only in meat, fish, and poultry. Vegetables and fruits are also part of the hypoglycemic diet and provide carbohydrates. Almost everything seems allowable on this hypoglycemic diet but in fact there are some critical foods that are not to be eaten.

Diet H—foods not allowed

Do not eat sugars and products containing sugars such as candy, soft drinks, cola drinks, grape juice, cakes, pastry, pancakes, waffles, jellies, jams, syrups, caramels, ice cream sundaes, etc., etc., etc.

Do not eat sugars.

Avoid all fruits that are canned in sugar syrups and dried fruits (drying the fruits concentrates the natural fruit sugars, so that they are almost as bad as refined sugar). During the first two weeks, avoid honey, after that perhaps a teaspoon or two is okay if not eaten all at once. After the first two weeks of this diet, one date per day is allowable. Avoid canned, smoked, prepared meats since most of these contain sugar. Read the labels very carefully.

Refined flour and starches are to be avoided in such products as spaghetti, noodles, and breads. If bread is an extremely important part of your diet, try to limit yourself to two slices per day. Corn is a source of easily assimilable sugars and starches and should be avoided, as well as potatoes, rice, sweet potatoes, and yams.

If you can stay away from the above foods, and be particularly alert for highly refined starch products and those containing sugar, you should start to feel better within several days of following this regimen.

DIET A—the allergic diet

Stop eating all dairy products, eggs, or products containing eggs or dairy products.

This diet is extremely straightforward. Stop eating all dairy products, eggs, or products containing eggs or dairy products. It's that simple. Let me give you the rationale for following this particular elimination diet.

Among the first foods that we receive after birth (with the exclusion of mother's milk) is cow's milk. For thousands of years people have been drinking cow's milk, and it is with this justification that cows are called the foster mother of humankind. There is reason to believe, however, that the infant's immunological system that prevents allergic reactions may not be fully developed at the time it first receives cow's milk. This is why allergy reactions to milk and dairy products are extremely common. Next to milk, allergic reactions to eggs are most common. By eliminating both of these, the chances are very good that if you have a food allergy at all, it will be taken care of through this plan. Stay on the diet for as long as it takes to adequately test its effects. (I will have more to say on this in the next section.)

Here are some hints to help you stay on the milk- and egg-free diet. Read the ingredients on the labels of products before you eat them. You might be surprised at the prevalence of milk and eggs in the variety of foods that you eat. Keep in mind that *sodium caseinate* and *whey* are milk products. Avoid many breads since they contain eggs or dairy products (although the following breads probably contain no milk or eggs—rye, italian, and french bread).

Many foods to which you might be allergic could be the cause of your headaches. It is best to see your doctor and/or allergist on this problem. In the absence of a medical diagnosis or evaluation of your allergy, the above diet is recommended.

DIET T—the tyramine-free and low chemical reaction diet

The tyramine-free, low chemical reaction diet is a rather easy one to follow. It includes a list of foods that must be avoided at all costs. These foods are known to contain tyramine and related chemical substances that can directly influence the occurrence of vasoconstrictions and vasodilations involved in migraine headaches.

Tyramine is a chemical which can directly influence the opening and closing of arteries, and under the right conditions can precipitate a migraine headache in individuals who are susceptible. There are two other substances which also can lead to headaches. The first of these is alcohol. In general, alcohol is a vasodilator, therefore, any type of alcoholic beverage when taken at the wrong time (particularly after there has been a sustained period of vasoconstriction) might bring on a headache. There are other contents of alcoholic beverages which could produce additional problems for the migraine headache sufferer. Alcoholic beverages contain more than just pure alcohol; it is these other substances which give them their distinctive tastes. Aromatic amines give wine its distinctive flavor. One of these is histamine which is known to directly affect vasoconstriction and vasodilation. Histamine is found particularly in red wines, hence it is not uncommon to find migraine patients who avoid red wines, but who drink the whites. Therefore, it appears that the migraine patient has to be extremely cautious when choosing and consuming alcohol. If you must drink, it is probably best to restrict your drinking to vodka, which is essentially pure alcohol, and of course, it should be consumed at a slow rate with water or with some other mixer.

Another chemical trigger is monosodium glutamate, or MSG. MSG is a chemical that is added to food to enhance flavor. It is extremely common in Chinese restaurants, although most restaurants probably use it in some of their dishes. MSG is often used in foods that are prepared some time before they are served, such as soups, stews, salad dressings, etc. For some individuals, MSG is such a potent producer of headaches, their headaches are called the "Chinese restaurant syndrome." MSG can be avoided by requesting that it not be added to food you eat (if made to order).

I'm going to add one other chemical trigger which was mentioned by Doctor J. B. Brainard in his book on migraine headaches. He found that many of his patients suffered migraine headaches after they ingested a sudden salt load. How the ingestion of a large amount of salt can produce a headache is not well understood, but it is related to the notion that the entire vascular system is influenced by the ingestion of salt. It is very easy to eat a large amount of salt in a short period of time: crackers, pretzels, potato chips, hors d'oeuvres, or just using excessive amounts of salt to flavor your food.

The diet for eliminating tyramine is given below. Carry the list with you and avoid these foods for a long enough period of time to determine whether or not your headaches have either disappeared or reduced in frequency. Later I will discuss in more detail how long this diet should be followed.

Avoid the following:

all ripened cheeses (cottage cheese is okay)
yogurt
avocados, bananas, citrus fruits, canned figs
onions
sudden salt load (crackers, salty snacks, ham, etc.)
pickled herring, anchovies
fermented sausage (bologna, salami, pepperoni, aged beef)
chicken livers, port, dried fish
nuts
navy, lima, fava beans
freshly baked bread
yeast extracts
red wine, sherry, beer (limited alcohol consumption is okay)
caffeine (coffee, tea, cola drinks)
chocolate, cocoa
MSG

How long do you stay on the diet?

The basic approach is one of experimentation. First, try a diet to see if it has a beneficial effect. If it is beneficial, I then recommend "challenging," which is explained below. If the first diet you try is not effective, then try one of the other diets (if appropriate). If none of the diets is effective and you have consulted with your doctor, then foods probably do not play a role in your headaches. In order to use this experimental approach, it is important that you regularly use biofeedback, Medlax, assertiveness, reanalysis of SADs, etc., while you try the diet.

The number of days or weeks that you stay on the diet varies from patient to patient and depends on the usual rate at which you experience migraine pain. If you get less than one headache per month, then it probably will be necessary for you to stay on this diet for a couple of months to find out if it is effective. If you get two or three headaches every two weeks, then it's probably sufficient to stay on the diet for a two-week period. I would recommend, however, that the diet be tried at least two weeks even if you get headaches on a daily basis. It generally takes at least two weeks for your body to readjust to the elimination of these foods and show a settling down of your artery reactions.

Challenging

After you have found a diet that reduces migraine pain, you can begin challenging. Challenging is the process by which you can determine how much and which type of foods can be tolerated before you again begin to experience headache symptoms. Whatever diet you have found to be effective (when used in combination with the control of other sources of vasoconstriction) can be challenged by adding one food or type of food to determine if it will produce headaches. The rate at which you experiment by adding foods depends again on how frequently your headaches used to occur. If you had a headache once a month, then after you have eliminated your headaches, let's say, by using Diet A for at least two months to assess its effectiveness, you could then start eating a small amount of eggs for two months to ascertain if your headaches recur. If they do, then you have to back off completely or reduce the amount of eggs that you eat.

The same principle holds true for the other diets. That is, very cautiously and gradually reintroduce one of the foods in the "avoided list" and find out if symptoms recur. By challenging, you can eventually determine the diet best suited for your individual needs.

Staying on the diet

If you have never dieted before, you are now going to be confronted with the difficulties encountered in attempting to control lifelong habits. The foods that we eat are very much a part of us, and it is usually difficult to change such basic behaviors. I leave you to your own devices to stay on your diet, but let me give you a few suggestions.

First, recognize that you might break the diet from time to time no matter how diligent you are. It is important to recognize and accept this fact. Research on habit control has shown that individuals who have difficulty controlling certain addictions, like alcohol, coffee, drugs, cigarettes, etc., do okay until they have a single relapse—a single cigarette, a glass of wine. Then they lose all hope that they will be able to shake the habit and return to their former heavy usage. If you can be prepared for these "relapses" by recognizing that they are normal and are bound to occur, you can start again with renewed efforts to maintain the diet.

Second, look at the diet as an experiment that will end in a few weeks' time. If you like a certain food that is no longer on your diet, it can be quite dismal to think about never having that food again. This is especially true since you're not even sure that the food is implicated in your migraine headaches. If you see your diet as simply a short experiment to gain information about your own body's reactions and what it takes to control headaches, not that you are starting a lifelong diet of any type, it will be much easier to remain on the diet.

Third, keep in mind that with this experimental diet you are making a major step toward the eradication of migraine pain. Once you have completed the experiment you will have another tool at your disposal to combat your headaches. Whether or not you use this tool, i.e., not eating certain foods, will be a choice that you can make at any time, just as you can choose whether or not to do the Medlax, reanalyze SADs, etc., and reduce headache pain. In the final analysis, it will be up to you whether avoiding a certain food or taking time out to do important vasodilation exercises are worth the potential avoidance of a headache.

Fourth, tell as many people as possible about your diet and how long you intend to stay on it. Try to enlist their support and encouragement.

Fifth, don't tempt yourself. Try to get rid of foods that are not on your diet. Don't leave them on shelves or in the refrigerator, where you'll be confronted with them at your weakest moment. Again, it's important to enlist the support of your family and living mates if possible.

Sixth, if you have kept on the diet, liberally reward yourself. That is, every day or every other day, give yourself a treat of special approved foods. This rewarding technique is especially critical if your family continues to eat foods not on your diet and you must see others consuming your favorites. Buy a special serving of cracked crab, for example, that is just for you and not to be shared with anyone else. This special reward is given because of the deprivations you have suffered.

Seventh, if you are sick or weak, forget about the diet until you have recovered. It's difficult enough to deal with illness without having to struggle with an experimental diet at the same time.

Eighth, if you are eating out, it may be necessary to give special instructions to the waitress or waiter. It's best not to overexplain why you are making your request, simply say, for example, "I do not want any butter on my potatoes." Similarly, when eating at a friend's house, if you let them know your dietary requirements, they are usually more than happy to accommodate you.

Finally, as special insurance, eat foods that are on your diet before you go to a restaurant or a party where you will be confronted with temptations that are difficult to resist. This pre-eating will help you considerably to stay on your diet.

APPENDIX

MEDICATION
AND THE TREATMENT
OF MIGRAINE

It may seem peculiar to some readers that a psychologist would include an appendix on medication in a book emphasizing nondrug approaches. The use of the Medlax and the biotic band, reanalysis of SADs, assertiveness, diet, etc., are all procedures for helping the migraine sufferer to gain control of his or her headaches without the use of medication, or at least without having to increase the amount of medication currently being used. This does not mean, however, that medication cannot play a role (perhaps, even a major role) in the overall treatment and control of your migraine headaches. One of the notions that I have tried to convey in this book is that migraine headache is a complicated disorder and that its control and treatment is equally complex and varies from person to person.

Individual differences in treatment also applies to the use of medication in the control of migraine. For example, some patients are able to control their pain just by doing their biofeedback experiments as suggested in chapter 2, whereas others are only helped by a combination of dietary and Medlax procedures. Similar differences are found in the usefulness of medication. For some individuals, the use of medication is an adequate and sometimes excellent solution to their pain problems. For other people, the medication may produce more side effects and problems than benefits and hence is not a satisfactory solution. Nevertheless, I would like to emphasize that medication *for some patients* will reduce or eliminate their pain and have minimal side effects. Furthermore, the use of the medication may not place the individual at unjustifiable risk. Since there are medications that meet these requirements of acceptability for *some* patients and since migraine headache is an exceptionally painful and disabling disorder, I recommend that you consider using medication (along with other methods outlined in this book) but that you discuss this with your doctor. Nearly all of the medications discussed in this appendix require a doctor's prescription. This requirement is for your protection since your particular medical history and physical makeup must be taken into account before these medications can be safely used. Of course, it would be best if you could control your headaches and ease the pain without the use of drugs. But, for some patients, a combination of the techniques described in this book and some medication (as prescribed by your doctor) is a perfectly satisfactory way of achieving adequate control over the pain.

Most migraine sufferers are already using medication prescribed by their doctor. If you are one of these people you probably bought this book because you are not completely satisfied with the effectiveness of the medication and/or because the side effects strongly detract from whatever benefits you may receive. Further, some patients have been told by their doctors that they are taking too much medication and should cut back on the frequency and the dosage levels they are using. If you fall into this category, then your interest in this book might well derive from your search for an alternative means of controlling your headaches. Whatever your category, I think that all migraine patients can benefit by understanding more about the medicines used in treating their headaches.

Migraine patients seem to have a peculiar attitude about medication. This became apparent to me during a midmorning break at one of my workshops for migraine headache sufferers. There in the men's room I saw fifteen or twenty workshop participants trying to hide the fact that they were taking medicine, opening the bottles with their backs toward me and trying to swallow their medication in an unobtrusive way. For some reason, migraine headache sufferers seem unique among medical patients in their degree of shame and guilt over taking medicine for this very disabling problem. Let me address this guilt by pointing out that you suffer from excruciating pain that very few individuals can appreciate unless they themselves have the same problem. The use of medication and any other type of useful treatment is more than justified by the relief from the disability and discomfort that these headaches cause.

Another reason for including this appendix is that certain new medications have been developed which can be quite effective for some people. You may have been suffering from these headaches for ten, twenty, thirty, forty or more years. Initially, when you first had them the general pattern was frequent visits to the doctor and a variety of medications were tried. If these medications were effective for you and did not produce side effects or dangerous reactions, then it is unlikely that you would be reading this book. However, after all appropriate medicines had been tried and not worked for you, your doctor may have said, "You're just going to have to learn to live with the problem." You might have just done that—learned to endure the pain—and no longer consult your physician about the headaches. This appendix is to alert you to the new medications. You can then discuss them with your doctor to see if they would be appropriate in your case.

Finally, this appendix affords me the opportunity to touch on the biochemistry of migraine headaches. By the biochemistry of migraine, I mean the presence in the body of certain chemical substances which probably play an important role in the cause of your headaches. Although the role is quite complex, this simplified explanation will give you some notion about the "chemical" causes of migraine headaches. As you now know, a headache is brought on by the two-phase reaction of arteries in the head. The first reaction is vasoconstriction which eventually leads to a compensatory vasodilation.

We know that the initial constriction of arteries is accompanied by and perhaps even caused by an excessively high concentration of *serotonin* in the blood stream. This biochemical, which incidentally everybody has, produces vasoconstriction by acting directly on the arterial wall. It is also known that the serotonin levels in the blood stream will then suddenly drop, and the blood vessels then dilate, producing the pain of a migraine headache. The major causes of the initial high levels of serotonin in your blood stream are known to be stress and foods. The subsequent fall in serotonin levels is due to a compensatory reaction of the body. Hence, the techniques described in this book—biofeedback, Medlax, diet, SADs, etc.—are designed to block this initial increase in serotonin, thus preventing or reversing vasoconstriction which is the first phase of your headache.

Throughout this book, I have emphasized that there are changes in the arteries which must be reckoned with in order to do something about migraine headaches. In considering the biochemistry— the level of serotonin in the bloodstream—it is possible to say that the techniques discussed in this book affect arteries by directly changing one's blood chemistry. Although it may seem farfetched that Medlax can actually change the chemical composition of the blood, numerous experimental studies indicate that relaxation-based techniques have precisely this effect.

As an interesting sidelight, I would like to point out that migraine headache sufferers are probably born with a propensity for excessively high blood levels of serotonin. Studies show that the blood of migraine sufferers is different from that of nonheadache patients. This difference in your blood makes you more likely to produce serotonin when under stress. In chapter 1, I mentioned that the tendency to have migraine headaches is probably inherited. Some medical researchers feel that the above mentioned difference in your blood might be inherited as well.

Many of the drugs that are used for migraine relief also affect the level of serotonin in the bloodstream (and elsewhere in the body) and tend to make these levels more normal. Therefore, it is possible to see how the combination of biofeedback, Medlax, SAD, reanalysis, diet, *and* perhaps the use of medication might control and provide relief from pain in a more effective way than is possible with any one or two of these factors by themselves.

Medications

I have classified the medications used in the treatment of migraine headaches into three categories: *analgesic* (pain relieving), *abortive*, and *prophylactic* (preventive). The newer types are primarily *prophylactic* (see tables 1, 2 and 3). While these categories do not include every medication in use, they do tend to cover the major ones.

Analgesic medications

Analgesic, or pain relieving, medications refer to those medicines which do nothing about the underlying causes of the pain itself—the dilation or constriction of arteries—but simply reduce the sensitivity of your pain receptors or your perception of pain. As you probably know, the feeling of pain is transmitted through special nerves whose only function is to let you know when pain is present. The use of an analgesic interferes with the pain receptors' ability to transmit impulses with your perception of the pain; thus one's experience of the pain is decreased. Although pain relievers can often play an important role in migraine headache relief, there is always the danger of overuse and habituation. By *habituation*, I refer to the possibility that over time more and more medication may be needed to produce the same pain-relief.

Abortive medications

The abortive drugs are those used when you can anticipate a headache or you know one is just getting underway, to prevent it from developing. The most common abortive medications are the ergot types (ergotamine, ergovine, etc.). These medications come in both capsule and pill form and are ingested orally. They are also available in inhaler, suppository, and injectable forms. Their primary mode of action is vasoconstriction. Some readers may be confused as to the benefits of this medication since vasoconstriction is the first phase of the two-phase response that leads to migraine pain.

Although exactly how ergot derivatives work is not known, it is suspected that they can prevent the pain of migraine by preventing the vasodilation phase itself. For many individuals, the use of an ergot-type medication at the first sign of a headache prevents the vasodilation which is just about to occur but the effect of the medication wears off very gradually in the hours immediately after it is ingested so that the vasoconstriction-vasodilation sequence is broken and the headache is aborted. For some persons, however, as the ergotamine effects wear off the onset of a headache is once again experienced. This "rebounding" has to do with the fact that the medication is really *producing* the first phase of the two-phase response leading to pain.

Many patients use ergotamine at dose levels and at frequencies that far exceed those prescribed by their physician. Ergotamine, like almost any medication, should only be used as directed. If you have been overusing this medication, it is highly recommended that you discuss with your physician how you can return to the prescribed dose. Some individuals who have negative reactions to ergotamine (stomach upset, dizziness, nausea, etc.) have found that similar vaso-constrictive medications not based on ergot compounds can be effective.

Prophylactic medications

The prophylactic medications, as contrasted with the abortive medications, are taken every day regardless of whether one feels a headache coming on. It is in the prophylactic category that new compounds are being used. One of the original abortive medications was Sansert (methysergide), which was known to interfere with the action of serotonin on arterial walls. Sansert is generally prescribed for six months to one year at a time, after which it is recommended that the patient take a "vacation" from the medication. If you have been taking Sansert on a regular basis and have not had a vacation from the use of the drug for some time, discuss this with your doctor to see if it is applicable in your case.

There are two new medications in this category that show promise. The first of these medications is called propranolol (Inderal, Inderide), and like all prophylactic medications, it is taken on a daily basis whether or not you feel a headache coming on. The use of propranolol in the treatment of migraine headache was discovered by accident. The drug was initially used for individuals who had suffered from heart attacks and was quite effective in preventing such individuals from suffering further heart attacks. In the initial clinical trials of this drug, a number of these patients who also regularly suffered from migraine headaches discovered that the drug eliminated their headaches. Since that time a number of studies found that some migraine sufferers do get relief when propranolol is taken on a regular basis.

A second new type of medication is the tricyclic antidepressants. Tricyclic antidepressant medications were given to migraine headache sufferers for two reasons. First, this medication was found to be useful in another acutely painful disorder called trigeminal neuralgia. Second, it was observed that migraine headache sufferers are frequently in a depressed state. While some researchers have noted that migraine headaches are caused by depression, it has been my experience that exactly the opposite is true—the depression is caused by the migraine headaches. I have seen patients who have gained control of their migraine headaches and correspondingly eliminated their depression. Regardless of the original rationale, it has been found that these medications can be helpful for some migraine patients. Like all medications, there are side and adverse effects. Tricyclics are one of those drugs, however, for which the benefits may not appear until you have given the drugs an adequate trial. If you and your doctor decide to try a tricyclic antidepressant, you should be prepared for the fact that there may be some immediate unpleasant side effects that need to be tolerated before benefits can be adequately assessed.

This appendix on migraine medication provides a general overview. It is important to keep in mind that dosage, side effects, and advisability of use are highly specific. Before any medication is used or before its dose level is changed, it is crucial that you consult with your doctor. Many of the medications described here, and others commonly used by migraine patients, should not be stopped suddenly. If you feel that you can get along without your medication because you have been using the techniques in this book and your headaches are under control, it is very important that you do not discontinue your medication abruptly without discussing this fully with your doctor.

TABLE 1   ANALGESICS

BRAND NAME(S)	CHEMICAL (GENERIC) NAME	ACTIONS/SIDE EFFECTS
Demerol, Dolosal	Meperdine hydrochloride	Central nervous system depressant, analgesic and sedative. May be habit-forming.
Darvon	Propoxyphene	Similar to codeine, analgesic. May be habit-forming.
Tylenol	Acetaminophen	Decreases activity of brain and relieves pain. Causes peripheral vasodilation.
	Aspirin	Analgesic, believed to prevent release of serotonin into blood stream.
	Phenacetin	Similar to Tylenol.
Codeine		Analgesic, may be habit-forming.
Percodan	Oxycodone in combination with aspirin, phenacetin and caffeine.	Similar to codeine; caffeine produces vasoconstriction.
Tylenol #1,2,3,4 or Empirin #2,3,4	Combinations with codeine.	May be habit-forming.
Fiorinol	Combination of butalbital aspirin, phenacetin, caffeine	Butalbital is a barbiturate which has analgesic effects and can enhance the effectiveness of the other analgesics in this compound. Can be habit-forming.

TABLE 2 ABORTIVE MEDICATIONS

BRAND NAME(S)	CHEMICAL NAME	ACTIONS/SIDE EFFECTS
Gynergen, Ergomar, Ergostat, Medihaler-Ergotamine, Femergin	Ergotamine tartrate	Tends to cause vasoconstriction, but also acts in a more general way to interfere with vascular system reactions.
Cafergot	Combination of ergotomine and caffeine	The caffeine increases the vasoconstrictive effect of ergotomine.
Periactin	Cyproheptadine hydrochloride	An antihistamine; also blocks action of serotonin.
Midrin	Combination of isomethep-tene, dichloraphenazone, and acetaminophen.	Blocks neural activity, affecting arteries. Sometimes used when ergot types are not effective or not tolerated by patient.

TABLE 3 PROPHYLACTIC MEDICATIONS

BRAND NAME(S)	CHEMICAL NAME	ACTIONS/SIDE EFFECTS
Sansert	Methysergide	Blocks the action of serotonin and prevents release of histamines, also affects central nervous system that regulates vascular reactions. Drug free "holidays" are recommended about every six months.
Elavil, Endep	Amitriptyline	Originally used for its antidepressant effects, has other effects of benefit to migraine sufferers by affecting the nerve pathways that lead to vasoconstriction.
Inderal	Propranolol	Believed to block vasodilation phase of headache. May not affect aura but can prevent or reduce pain phase.
	Lithium carbonate	For cyclical or cluster migraines (see amitriptyline above).

INDEX

PERSONAL HANDWARMING DIARY

Name: _____

DATE	TIME OF DAY	TYPE ACTIVITY B = BIOFEEDBACK M = MEDLAX O = OTHER	FINGER TEMPERATURE (BEFORE HANDWARM ATTEMPT)		FINGER TEMPERATURE (AFTER HANDWARM ATTEMPT)		NOTES
			GUESS*	ACTUAL	GUESS*	ACTUAL	

* The "Guess" column is explained in chapter 4.
© 1979, 1983 by R. J. Kohlenberg, Ph.D.

Replacement Biotic Bands are available for $6.50 each. Send check or money order and a stamped, self-addressed envelope to:

Biofeedback and Stress Management Clinic
Lakeview Medical
3216 N.E. 45th Place
Seattle, Washington 98105

PERSONAL HANDWARMING DIARY

Name: _____

DATE	TIME OF DAY	TYPE ACTIVITY B = BIOFEEDBACK M = MEDLAX O = OTHER	FINGER TEMPERATURE (BEFORE HANDWARM ATTEMPT)		FINGER TEMPERATURE (AFTER HANDWARM ATTEMPT)		NOTES
			GUESS*	ACTUAL	GUESS*	ACTUAL	

*The "Guess" column is explained in chapter 4.

PERSONAL HANDWARMING DIARY

Name: _____

DATE	TIME OF DAY	TYPE ACTIVITY B = BIOFEEDBACK M = MEDLAX O = OTHER	FINGER TEMPERATURE (BEFORE HANDWARM ATTEMPT)		FINGER TEMPERATURE (AFTER HANDWARM ATTEMPT)		NOTES
			GUESS*	ACTUAL	GUESS*	ACTUAL	

*The "Guess" column is explained in chapter 4.

© 1979, 1983 by R. J. Kohlenberg, Ph.D.